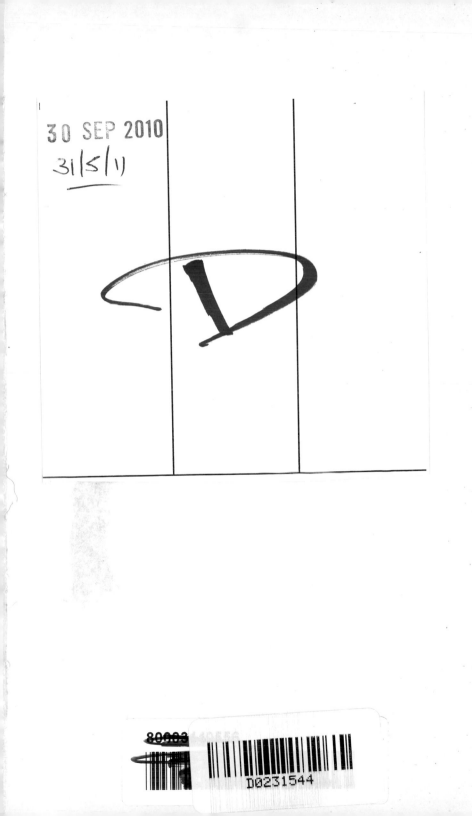

Tapping for Life

Janet Thomson MSc

HAY HOUSE

Australia • Canada • Hong Kong • India
South Africa • United Kingdom • United States

Northamptonshire Libraries & Information Services DD

First ~~published and distributed in the United Kingdom by:~~
Hay House UK ~~Ltd,~~ Rd, London W10 5BE. Tel.: (44) 20 ~~8962~~ 2 1230;
~~(44) 20 8962 1239. www.hayhouse.co.uk~~

Publis ~~hed and distributed in the United States of America by:~~
Hay House, In ~~c., PO Box 5100, Carlsbad, CA 92018-5100. Tel.: (1) 760~~ 31 7695
or (800) 654 5 ~~126; Fax: (1) 760 431 6948 or (800) 650 5115. www.hayhouse.com~~

Askews

Hay H ~~ouse Australia Ltd, 18/36 Ralph St, Alexandria NSW 201~~
Tel.: (61) ~~2 9669 4299; Fax: (61) 2 9669 4144. www.hayhouse.com.au~~

Publis ~~hed and distributed in the Republic of South Africa by:~~
Ha ~~y House SA (Pty), Ltd, PO Box 990, Witkoppen 2068.~~
~~Tel./Fax: (27) 11 467 8904. www.hayhouse.co.za~~

Published and distributed in India by:
Hay House Publishers India, Muskaan Complex, Plot No.3, B-2, Vasant Kunj,
New Delhi – 110 070. Tel.: (91) 11 4176 1620; Fax: (91) 11 4176 1630.
www.hayhouse.co.in

Distributed in Canada by:
Raincoast, 9050 Shaughnessy St, Vancouver, BC V6P 6E5.
Tel.: (1) 604 323 7100; Fax: (1) 604 323 2600

© Janet Thomson, 2010

The moral rights of the author have been asserted.

The author of this book does not dispense medical advice or prescribe the use of any technique as a form of treatment for physical or medical problems without the advice of a physician, either directly or indirectly. The intent of the author is only to offer information of a general nature to help you in your quest for emotional and spiritual wellbeing. In the event you use any of the information in this book for yourself, which is your constitutional right, the author and the publisher assume no responsibility for your actions.

A catalogue record for this book is available from the British Library.

ISBN 978-1-84850-188-1

Printed and bound in Great Britain by TJ International, Padstow, Cornwall.

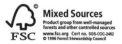

Mixed Sources
Product group from well-managed
forests and other controlled sources
www.fsc.org Cert no. SGS-COC-2482
© 1996 Forest Stewardship Council

This book is dedicated to Roger Callahan, without whose brilliance many thousands of people across the world would still be experiencing unnecessary suffering. On behalf of all those who have been set free ... and all those who will be as a result of your amazing discoveries ... thank you.

Also to Richard Bandler and John Grinder, who revolutionized psychological therapies with their insatiable curiosity and determination to challenge existing thinking.

All three of these incredible people were brave enough to challenge the 'establishment' and had an unswerving belief that change is possible and it doesn't have to be painful. Luckily for all of us, they were right.

Contents

Foreword

In *Tapping for Life*, Janet Thomson has done a masterful job of combining her real-life experiences, years of education in exercise and nutrition, and her skill in tho application of a powerful healing modality, along with her knowledge of NLP, into a simple straightforward manual for, as she so eloquently states, self-empowerment.

In *Tapping for Life*, the reader learns how TFT was discovered and has developed over the last 30 years. Janet clearly explains the difference between TFT and the many tapping therapies that have evolved from this highly effective modality. She not only captures the essence of why they all work to varying degrees but why TFT is so much more effective.

Janet is creative and unique in her ability to explain the basis of how TFT and our negative emotions operate. Her explanation of the meridians as 'emotional information highways' paints a clear picture helping the reader to understand a complicated theory. She also clearly explains the three levels of TFT protocols – algorithm, diagnostic and Voice Technology (VT) – and their comparative successes.

Her focus on some of the most important concepts and procedures, such as psychological reversal and the use of the voltmeter, provide the reader with immediate and objective measurable tools for healing. The cases give clear examples, such as pain, trauma, guilt, weight loss, etc, that are easy for everyone to relate to.

Janet is an approved TFT algorithm level trainer and combines her excellent teaching skills, excitement and knowledge in her trainings. She has done an excellent job of creating positive media attention and we are proud to have her as a representative for TFT in the UK.

Roger J. Callahan PhD
Founder and Developer of Thought Field Therapy
Chairman of the Board, Association for Thought Field Therapy

Joanne M. Callahan MBA
President, Callahan Techniques, Ltd
President, ATFT Foundation

Acknowledgements

Synchronicity is a beautiful thing. I was at my PC one day, working on a book proposal, and had just called Hay House Publishers to ask to whom I needed to send it. I was told that they were not accepting any more proposals at the present time. I was disappointed, as Hay House was my first choice because I am huge fan of Louise Hay and of the Hay House catalogue and the kind of titles they represent. As I hung up, a friend of mine called Nicole Barber Lane rang to tell me that she and her husband Paul were listening to Chris Evans' Radio 2 show and he was talking about how to stop cravings, and as I had taught them both how to eliminate cravings with Thought Field Therapy, they said I should ring up the show. Unable to get through, I sent a text, if only because I knew Nicole would check on me to make sure I had! The next day I had a call from the producer, and that evening I was on the show talking about and demonstrating for listeners the awesome power of TFT. Chris Evans was charming and very open to this great technique, which he could actually see working, and as a result very many listeners learned about TFT and began to benefit from it personally. Also listening was a senior member of staff at Hay House, who thought it would make a great basis for a book. One lunchtime meeting later … and here is the result. This book was meant to be written, possibly just so that *you* could read it and benefit from it.

Now *that's* synchronicity.

Janet

A New Present

It is the human situation to meet the present with interpretations of the past.

The meaning of the present is to allow us to leave the past and see the NOW in its own right.

Experience will soon become your past and a foundation for a new and present future.
Virginia Satir

Introduction

After working with individual clients and groups for over 25 years as a personal trainer, I got pretty good at helping people change their bodies. I'd had years of academic study and attained a Master's Degree in Exercise and Nutrition Science, combined with *real life* practical experience as both a consultant for a top national slimming group and running my own small chain of fitness clubs, along with an impressive track record as a presenter, author and 'trainer of trainers'. In spite of all of this, I was dissatisfied. I felt I could do better. Why? Because in front of me were all these people who were transformed physically, yet they still carried all the negative emotions and feelings they had had when they were big. All of the sadness, trauma or anxiety that caused them to overeat in the first place was still there. I began to search for effective ways to help these people, and soon learned that overeating was usually a symptom of something much deeper that had not been resolved.

Over the years I heard so many heartbreaking stories of years of depression, abuse, anxiety and immense sadness, I knew I had to find some way to *fix the head* before I fixed the body.

After spending almost two years training as a Life Coach, I learned some techniques that were helpful, but not quick enough for my impatient mind. Then I heard about Neuro-Linguistic Programming (NLP), a system for understanding *how your brain works* and how to bring about fast, effective, permanent change. I felt that at last I was on the right track.

I enrolled on an NLP Practitioners course and awaited it with excitement and optimism.

Life has a funny way of kicking us up the backside at the appropriate moment and teaching us something we need to know, whether you call it fate, God, coincidence, or whatever your belief system. These lessons are not always easy to learn. Two days before the course was due to begin, I faced a significant family trauma. What it was is not important; in true stiff-upper-lip British fashion I pulled myself together and went away to the course.

Within the first 30 minutes we were being asked to 'think a happy thought' so we could 'anchor' it and be able to access it at any time. I was in such a bad place I just could not think up any happy thoughts at all. I went to the back of the room to tell one of the assistants I was going home, that I was not in the right place to do this training. She sat me down, asked me to think about the problem – she didn't want all the details, which was good because I was in no fit state to talk. All I had to do, she said, was think about it myself. She then began to tap me, gently, tapping various points around my face and on my hands, as I sat there sobbing. I was mystified, but too upset to protest. Literally within the first two minutes I began to feel like a huge weight was falling away from me. The crying stopped; she continued to tap and I felt with amazement the trauma literally collapse and disappear. I still had the knowledge of what had happened, of course, but now I could think about it without the angst and pain I had been experiencing just minutes earlier.

That was my first introduction to Thought Field Therapy (TFT). I knew right then that this was a technique I *had* to learn, and from that moment on both TFT and NLP have been a crucial part of my work, both in my own life and in helping others. Without experiencing my own trauma at exactly that time, I might never have been introduced to TFT in such a powerful way.

Now I want to share its amazing power with YOU.

How would you feel if you had, quite literally at your fingertips, the means to collapse any negative feeling or emotion that has been holding you back? Read on.

Part 1
All About Thought Field Therapy

What Is 'Tapping'?

The concept of 'Tapping' was created by the brilliant Dr Roger Callahan. Dr Callahan has an impressive academic record which includes being an Associate Professor and a Research Clinical Psychologist; he is currently a Fellow of the American Academy of Psychotherapists Treating Addiction.

The story begins in 1981. Dr Callahan was working in his clinic, and had an appointment with a client named Mary. Mary had a lifelong fear of water. Her phobia was so bad she could not go out in the rain, or even take a full bath. They had been working together for some time and Dr Callahan had used every method he knew possible; being a specialist in treating phobics, he had made some progress, if you could call it that, in that Mary could now stand more pain than she ever thought possible, by allowing herself to be near water. However, doing so caused her great anguish. Dr Callahan was frustrated by this and, like all great minds, he had been seeking answers elsewhere as to how he could help Mary and others like her. These enquiries had included investigations into applied kinesiology (a system of testing the muscles to gauge feedback on the body's functioning), and also the meridians (as used in acupuncture and Traditional Chinese Medicine). We will learn more about meridians later.

While working with Mary on this particular day, Dr Callahan asked her to tap the area under her eye – linked to the stomach meridian, and this is where Mary was experiencing her anxiety. While tapping she was asked to think about water. Thinking about water wasn't difficult for

Mary, as they were outside, fairly near to a swimming pool. The concept of being 'in the thought field' is critical to TFT, as we will discover. After a few seconds of tapping, Mary said 'It's gone!', meaning the feeling of anxiety and terror in her body. She then walked over to the pool, leaving a bewildered Dr Callahan behind her, now more anxious than she. She called out to him, 'Don't worry, I know I can't swim.' Mary's phobia had vanished completely – years of terror gone in just a few seconds.

That night there was a terrible storm, which up until then would have brought about an anxiety attack for Mary. Instead she got in her car and drove to the beach, got out and walked to the water's edge to watch the storm. No anxiety whatsoever. The phobia had gone.

Dr Callahan was delighted by this result, and of course for the next phobic who walked through the door he tried the same technique. This time, however, there was not the same dramatic result. However, Callahan had witnessed the power of 'Tapping' (then called Callahan Techniques) and knew he was on the threshold of discovering a genuine method of treatment which could prove beneficial beyond compare within the field of psychological therapies.

This is exactly what proved to be the case, as he studied and developed this method over the next few years. In fact he is still working hard and developing it today several decades later, despite being a youthful 80-something years young.

Dr Callahan's path over the next few years was not an easy one. The orthodox medical profession criticized him for using the word 'cure', even attempting legal action to stop him. Traditional psychotherapy just could not conceive of 'eliminating' a problem outright. Traditional thinking had been that patients had to 'learn to live with it'. Phrases like 'feel the fear and do it anyway' were commonplace. How much better, though, to *eliminate* the fear and do it anyway?! Dr Callahan's methods fitted about as well as a square peg into a round hole when compared to traditional methods, not least because his methods worked so well. In her excellent book *The Field*, Lynn McTaggart says:

> *'To be revolutionary in science today is to flirt with professional suicide. Much as the field purports to encourage experimental freedom, the entire structure of science, with its highly competitive grant system coupled with the publishing and peer review system, largely depends upon individuals conforming to the accepted world view. The system tends to encourage professionals to carry out experimentation whose purpose is to confirm the existing view of things.'*

I feel this could have been written specifically about Dr Callahan. Thankfully for all of us, he persevered, often at great personal and professional cost, to develop this amazing therapy so that people just like you and me can use it quickly and effectively, and reap the benefits.

Since that time in 1981, others have used the 'Tapping' principle – and renamed it. Gary Craig, who worked and trained with Dr Callahan for some time, now uses Tapping under the heading Emotional Freedom Technique (EFT). You will learn more about the differences between EFT and TFT later on, but in essence TFT works with a number of specific diagnosed points, depending on the emotion or feeling you want to eliminate, whereas EFT uses all the points all the time, alongside phrases spoken out loud. As you will see, this process is unnecessarily long and involved.

Dr Callahan's system is probably the most underrated psychological treatment available. I believe this is because its simplicity almost beggars belief; people cannot understand how or why they can eliminate feelings that have held them back for years, maybe even decades, in just a few minutes – but they can.

Psychological Reversal

One crucial aspect of TFT, missing from most other 'adaptations' (including EFT) is Dr Callahan's discovery of a condition he terms 'psychological reversal' (PR). This is when your mind does the opposite of what you want it to; in practical terms this can mean putting the butter in the oven and the chicken in the fridge, putting something down and immediately forgetting to remember where you've put it. We can all relate to this! In fact, most of us are in and out of PR every day in some form or another, but, critically, PR can do more harm than just causing us to make simple errors: it can also prohibit healing and recovery from illness, and amplify negative emotions.

Try It for Yourself Right Now

Clearing or correcting PR takes literally seconds. You can start using this simple technique right now. This technique alone is worthy of ten seconds of your time several times a day, and can help with motivation, energy levels, concentration, self-esteem, removing negative thoughts and promoting physical health and healing. It is the single most powerful and possibly the most important component of TFT.

To clear or correct PR, you simply tap the side of your hand 15+ times, on the 'karate' spot.

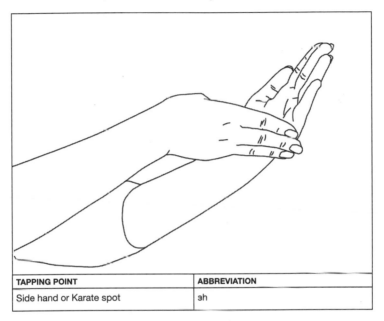

TAPPING POINT	ABBREVIATION
Side hand or Karate spot	sh

Get into the routine of doing this every time you wash your hands, whether you think you need it or not. If you are not in PR and you tap, it does no harm. It certainly does not put you into PR if you tap when you don't need to. Like all TFT methods, there are NO negative side effects whatsoever. You either need it and it works, or it does nothing.

Later on we'll learn how to test if you (or someone you are helping) is in PR.

The reason this is the first technique I am teaching you is that, as simple as it is, it's THE most important tapping point on the body.

The Benefits of Thought Field Therapy

Therapists and teachers of TFT, such as myself, continue to use TFT, alone or in combination with other techniques such as NLP. (I will tell you much more about NLP later.) While we may add our own touches to it, and incorporate it with other disciplines, the concept of TFT remains as Dr Callahan taught us.

Some of the main benefits of TFT as a treatment are that it's non-invasive, it can be self-administered and it does no harm. If you tap the wrong points, or do not use the techniques correctly, then you'll do yourself no harm. You get a positive result, or you get nothing. No nasty side effects, no pills to swallow, no need to spend hours talking about the problem. Remember, there are NO negative side effects whatsoever to TFT.

The difference between a skilled therapist who gets great resu lts (typically my own success rate is around 90 per cent) and an average therapist who gets around 70 per cent success (which is still pretty impressive!) is in *how* TFT is applied. The purpose of *Tapping for Life* is to teach YOU to become your own TFT Therapist, so that YOU can treat yourself by eliminating past traumas, curing phobias and anxiety, and regaining control of your life. There is almost no negative emotion that you cannot treat with TFT. It's both empowering and liberating. Read on.

Treating Trauma

TFT is now used all over the world, often in areas of great trauma. The Association of Thought Field Therapy (ATFT) has a Trauma Relief Committee (see Further Resources at the back of the book) which travels to places such as Rwanda, where practitioners work with orphans and survivors of genocide, with astonishing results, bringing emotional relief to people who have been through an unbelievable level of suffering.

And it's not just in war-torn areas where people are benefiting from TFT to remove traumatic experiences and emotions. Every day, TFT therapists are working with people just like you.

Now YOU can benefit personally from these simple techniques by using them on yourself.

In addition to removing negative emotions and feelings, you will also learn some valuable techniques to replace negative feelings with new, more positive ones. Often when clients come to see me, having suffered for years with anxiety or depression, they can be left with a void when the negative emotions have gone. It sounds crazy, perhaps, but some people get so used to feeling anxious that when you remove the anxiety they feel lost! We get used to what we know, even if we don't like it.

By understanding how your brain works, you can learn to think differently in order to get a different outcome. Behaviour patterns can be deleted and replaced with new, more beneficial ones. You will learn how to do this – and have fun in the process – later in the book. First, let's take a look at how TFT works.

How Does TFT Work?

The simple answer is: very well!

TFT is different from any other form of psychotherapy because it is, by design, diagnostic in terms of how it was developed. It actually *removes* the underlying causes that created the problem in the first place.

Initially, as you have heard with Mary's story, Dr Callahan first made his discovery that tapping specific points worked to rob negative emotions of their power. This is done using *sensory feedback*. In other words, he tried it and he saw it worked. Not all the time, initially, but often enough for him to know that, with refinement, TFT was potentially a very successful treatment.

Most other psychological approaches are based on theories of what should predictably work, based on known patterns of behaviour. Often therapists in other disciplines are taught that if a treatment is not working it is because the client is emotionally repressed. In TFT, if a treatment is not working it's probably because of one of four things:

1. **You are not in the 'thought field' (TF – more about this in the next chapter)**
2. **You are using the wrong tapping sequence (this sequence is also known as an *algorithm*)**
3. **You are Psychologically Reversed (i.e. in PR).**
4. **You are suffering from Individual Energy Toxins (IETs).**

More about all of these later in the book.

Although TFT does not work in every case, in approximately 80 per cent of cases, if these criteria are met, then the treatment is likely to be successful and the problem eliminated.

Diagnosis

Using reality-based observations, Dr Callahan began to develop a system of what is termed *causal diagnosis*. To help figure out the best treatment for a patient, he used diagnostic kinesiology (a method used by some chiropractors which tests muscle strength to detect disease and other problems). Ultimately he developed Voice Technology (VT), a method of voice analysis that identifies the exact tapping points to be used and the order in which they are to be tapped for a given problem.

During the 1980s, as these methods were being developed, Dr Callahan noticed that particular sequences were being diagnosed repeatedly for certain problems. For example, for anxiety he frequently found the following sequence being indicated: under eye – under arm – collarbone.

From these bespoke sequences came the algorithms commonly used today, which you will find later in this book.

Diagnostic TFT (TFT-Dx) and VT can be seen as 'bespoke', and are therefore tailored to a specific individual's unique problems and issues.

Algorithms, on the other hand, are 'off the shelf' sequences known to work for most people. That probably includes you!

Results

Ultimately, TFT can be judged by the successful results you can achieve when you use it correctly. One of its many advantages is that it does not require you to delve into your dim and distant past or to relive all your childhood memories, or for you to be identified as a personality 'type' which should fit into this or that category. There is absolutely no need for you to understand how or why you feel like you do. You just need to know *how* you feel, and hold that thought while you tap.

When I have a client who has a long-standing trauma – for example if they were abused as a child – there is no need for them to describe it to me in any great detail. They do not need to spend hours talking about it, trying to understand it or 'deal with it' in any way whatsoever, and they certainly don't need to learn to live with it. We simply identify the associated feelings – perhaps anger, resentment, rage, anxiety, fear; whatever the emotions, the client simply has to think about them for a few minutes while we tap the relevant points, and the emotions and feelings associated with the event collapse. The client is then able to think about the abuse, will still know it happened, but will not be able to access the previously debilitating emotions attached to the abuse. TFT does not erase the memory or the 'data' of the event, it simply collapses all emotional attachment or responses to it.

The best way for you to appreciate the awesome power of TFT is to begin to use it; as you learn the techniques described in this book, you'll experience for yourself the often profound changes that occur.

Keeping It Simple

Let's remove some of the more complex detail and look at the process in simple terms. You know that in your body 'things' are transported by fluids; you have approximately 5 litres of blood, for example, which transports oxygen, nutrients and many other substances to and from the cells. Your lymphatic system contains approximately 15 litres of fluid which removes toxins in order to prevent them from entering the bloodstream. We also have nerve cells that transport signals to and from our brains. All of these things are tangible; we can see them inside a human body through various means such as X-rays or scans, we know they are there and we can see how specifically they work. But we also have another, equally significant system: centuries ago our meridians were identified, located and began to be used in Traditional Chinese Medicine (TCM). From this came the well-established technique we know as acupuncture, in which needles are used at very specific points along the meridians in order to move energy, or *chi*. Although some modern sceptics continue to deny the existence of meridians, they are widely accepted as crucial for maintaining emotional and physical health, not just by alternative therapists but also by orthodox practitioners and clinicians. In some parts of the UK, acupuncture is available on the NHS. It's frightening to think that certain sectors of the medical establishment can dismiss over 3,000 years of effective Eastern practice while in the West many thousands of deaths occur each year as a direct result of medical errors and adverse reactions to drugs. TFT, for its part, is a non-invasive, non-clinical treatment with zero risk of death.

It can be helpful to think of meridians as emotional highways: imagine your meridians as a motorway network, transporting information throughout your body in an efficient, timely manner. In this sense they are 'emotional information highways',

When you experience an event or a trauma, it can be seen as the equivalent of several vehicles colliding on the motorway, causing information to be stuck in the accident hotspot. This hotspot becomes the cause of a subsequent problem, i.e. a traffic jam.

In TFT terms, these hotspots are called Perturbations (Ps). It is the Ps that are specifically responsible for transmitting all the negative thoughts subsequently associated with that particular event.

It is important to note, however, that these Ps transmit that specific information when you are 'in the thought field' – that is, when you are recalling the event. However, even when you are not in the thought field, the Ps contribute to your emotional 'barrel' (more of this on page 25), as they contain information about stored negative emotions.

When you are in the thought field *and the Perturbations are activated, the relevant points along the meridians can be tapped and the emotion eliminated.*

Different thoughts and events cause a different pattern of Perturbations, and each pattern requires the correct tapping sequence so that it is eliminated completely. I will explain more about how to tap the correct sequence as we go along.

As with a series of motorway collisions, once the vehicles (the Ps) are cleared, the negative thoughts they transmitted are no longer generated. All that remains is a memory that there was a problem, leaving only a 'benign' thought behind. You are likely to be able to talk about the event (should you want to) without the previous emotional tidal wave. You will be able to recall what happened, you will remember that it was unpleasant, but you will disassociate from any physical or emotional response.

>>>Jean's story

One of my first clients was a lovely woman named Jean. She was totally traumatized by the death of her mother, almost a year previously. Her grief was palpable. She couldn't function at work, was shutting out her husband and could not speak about her mum without completely breaking down. We tapped for the sadness over the loss, and the guilt she felt for not doing more to help her mum (which, as with most people in her position, was completely unjustified, as she had done all she practically could).

Within 30 minutes of treatment, Jean began to chat about her mum fondly and without crying. She found this amazing, as she had not been able to mention the word 'mum' without completely breaking down just half an hour earlier. After a little more tapping she was telling funny stories about her mum and laughing and remembering the good times – again something she had been unable to do for almost a year as she couldn't get past the grief and the memory of her mother's passing. Suddenly it was as if Jean got all her good memories of her mum back, and experienced a level of joy and connection to her mother's memory that literally transformed her. A few weeks later she called me to say it had been the anniversary of her mum's death, and she and the family had sat around and celebrated her life, and chatted about all the good times. Without TFT she would have been unable to attend this event, let alone participate and celebrate her mother's life.

What Is a Thought Field?

Just take a moment to recall your happiest ever memory: perhaps meeting someone special for the first time, the birth of a child, a time when you achieved something you were really proud of, the sense of achievement and independence you felt when you passed your driving test, a romantic moment, or any other time when you felt fantastic. After you have finished reading this paragraph, just close your eyes and bathe yourself in that memory: immerse yourself in the vision, see what you saw, allow your ears and mind to hear again the sounds you heard; smell the smells you smelled. Remember how it all felt – where in your body was the feeling? In your tummy, butterflies in your chest perhaps? Allow these positive emotions and recollections to flow through your body right now for the next minute or so ...

Notice how the memory is not 'just a thought' but a physiological experience, a fusion of mind and body working together as you relive the experience. Maybe you feel excited? Or relaxed? I don't know how good you feel, but you do.

Have you ever been in a room with someone who was literally 'exuding' positive energy? So much so that when you are near them (i.e. within their energy field) you cannot help but feel their positive energy? Unfortunately, the opposite is also true: some people are so efficient at transmitting negative thoughts that you can be 'infected' by their negative energy and you too begin to feel down when you are near them. These are not people you should choose to spend too much time with.

Thoughts Do Matter

We often underestimate the physical connection between a thought, which is ultimately a series of chemical processes, and its fundamental effect on us as a whole, physically, spiritually and emotionally. Just because we cannot see our energy field, does not mean it does not exist or affect us at a functional level.

Think about gravity for a moment: you can't see it, yet you *know* it's there, that it has properties and obeys certain predictable principles. If you drop something, it falls down to the ground, not up to the sky. When Isaac Newton first noticed the apple falling from the tree, he didn't need to 'see' gravity to investigate its effects.

If you were to do a handstand for 5 minutes, you would feel the physical effects as an increase in the pressure in your head as the blood flows to your brain, which has no means of pumping it back against the force of gravity. When you are upright, i.e. standing on your feet, you have a marvellous system of vessels and valves that push the blood back up through the body to the heart. Large leg muscles stimulate this action every time you move. We were definitely designed to stand on our feet and not on our heads!

After watching the apple fall to the ground, Isaac Newton began to investigate the force of gravity and its far-reaching effects. It's amazing, isn't it? A seemingly tiny yet supremely astute observation, something as simple as watching an apple fall from the tree (which people too numerous to mention must have witnessed before without a second thought) led to the discovery that the moon is held in place by the gravitational pull of the earth. Newton went on to create equations for calculating the effects of gravity, and to conclude that its force extends across the whole universe. Wow. Yet we can't see it.

In a not dissimilar way, a single thought or series of thoughts can have far-reaching effects and extend throughout your body's physiology at a cellular level, affecting, potentially, every part of us. Our thoughts *do* matter.

What Do Your Thoughts Do to You?

How often are we told that stress is a risk factor and contributes to health problems such as heart disease (that's dis-ease) and cancer? Yet we associate this more with our 'lifestyle' than with our actual thoughts.

Think of the words 'stress' and 'depression' as verbs (i.e., 'doing' words). In this sense you don't 'have' depression, you 'do' depression. It is not an illness in the sense that measles is something you 'have'; whatever you 'do', if you are infected you 'have' measles.

To be depressed you have to process feelings and day-to-day experiences in a certain way, think certain (negative) thoughts and adopt certain (negative) behaviours, physically and emotionally, that combine to create the state of depression. If you stopped doing these things in this way, you would stop being depressed. Of course I am not saying it is easy, and I do not want to trivialize the effects of depression in any way. The key question is *how* can you stop 'doing' depression?

What I and many other practitioners have found when working with clients is that, by using TFT, you can eliminate the *causes* of the behaviours and thoughts that make up the act of 'doing' depression and regain control of your life. You will learn these skills as you continue to read through this book.

Warning!
Never, ever underestimate the potentially devastating effects of your negative thoughts on your body.

Bruce Lipton PhD, a renowned cell biologist, investigated the effect that non-clinical factors, including our thoughts and emotions, have on our cells. In his brilliant book *The Biology of Belief*, he explains how human cells are much like computer cells, in that they can both be programmed by influences outside of the cell. He describes the human cell nucleus as simply a memory disk, and the DNA programmes as the hard drive. In your PC you can insert a disk and download new files or programmes; these programmes still work even when the disk is removed, as the programme has been 'absorbed' into the very workings of the cell.

Lipton discovered that the many receptors on the cell membrane deliver information that influences the cells' behaviour, much like a keyboard is used to type instructions into your PC. He coined the phrase 'magical membrane'; this magical membrane is strongly influenced by your thoughts and beliefs, which can literally change the biology of your cells, thereby affecting your emotional and physical well-being. In short – you become what you think.

The mind/body connection is in a constant state of dynamic and delicate balance.

Dr Masaru Emotos, a doctor of alternative medicine, author and researcher from Japan, has carried out and replicated several experiments demonstrating the power of our thoughts on water. We know that water adapts physically to its environment: we are all aware, of course, that water turns to ice crystals when it freezes and into steam when heated. What Emotos demonstrated was an extraordinary change in water when it was exposed to different thoughts and words. He showed that if specific negative thoughts and words are directed at water before it is frozen, then the shape of the ice crystals is very 'ugly'. In direct contrast, when positive thoughts are directed to water before freezing, crystals of quite beautiful shape and design are produced. You can find the many pictures and photographs of this research on the Internet or in Emotos' book, *Messages from Water*.

If you consider that as babies we are up to 78 per cent water and as adults approximately 65 per cent, and that every single metabolic reaction within our cells happens in a 'wet' environment, and then consider that your thoughts and emotions can have a dramatic effect on the molecular structure of 'you', then you have an indication of how important it is to eliminate negative thoughts and emotions for good emotional and physical health.

The Barrel Effect: When You've Reached the Limit of What You Can Take

We all have a limit, a threshold if you like, of exactly how much 'stuff' we can deal with before we react physically and/or emotionally in a negative way.

Imagine that inside of you is a barrel, and this barrel holds all the negative emotions and feelings that you have gathered throughout your life. Because bad 'stuff' happens to all of us, the contents of the barrel are, to a certain extent, transient; this means that some of the feelings and emotions that come into this barrel are temporary and are subsequently removed by your unconscious, creating a 'turnover'. Others, however, stay inside the barrel permanently. The barrel gets heavier and heavier and more and more full as we get older, and it gets harder and harder to carry on. A bit like a saucepan that bubbles over when it is too full, at some point a full barrel will start to crack and creak under the strain. If it bursts completely, we have total emotional meltdown.

Often people come to see me with a particular problem, perhaps for weight loss or even a simple phobia; once we start working together and they realize the power of TFT, they ask if they can 'get rid' of some other 'stuff' as well. As a result, I regularly treat people for something completely different to their original problem.

A good example of this is a client who initially wants to stop smoking or lose weight. Once you remove the stress, anxiety and fear, especially if they are based on past trauma, then the need to smoke to relieve anxiety, or to comfort-eat, is removed and as a result the clients often spontaneously stop smoking or overeating as they begin to feel more positive about themselves generally.

If your emotional barrel is full, exactly what it is full of may be irrelevant. In other words, if you fell off a horse when you were six years old and broke a leg, that may take up some room in your barrel. If your parents got divorced or you lost a parent, that would inevitably take up a significant area. If you suffered a broken heart as a young lover, that would take up a bit, and so on and so forth until the barrel was full. All that matters is that the barrel *is* full. There may or may not be any connection between the different events that fill the barrel; all of the 'things' in it can, without exception, major and minor, be removed using TFT.

You will have heard the phrase 'the straw that broke the camel's back'. This is exactly the same principle: when the barrel is about to burst, the slightest small thing, which normally would barely even evoke a response, can cause a powerful negative reaction out of all proportion to the actual event or deed. When this happens, you need to take action and empty that barrel. Even better, empty it *before* it gets too full!

> *Once you have learned how to literally tap your troubles away, you will have this skill at your disposal for life, and you need never experience the effects of 'barrel-bursting' again.*

Once the barrel has been emptied using TFT to remove the negative thoughts, and specifically the Perturbations (Ps) that cause the negative feelings, it becomes harder to 'do' depression. Once these Ps have been removed and the negative thoughts and feelings eliminated, we can use other techniques such as Neuro-Linguistic Programming (NLP) to reprogramme our brains to 'do' things differently, think different thoughts and choose different behaviours.

TFT and NLP work so well together in this way. TFT removes the negative feelings, and NLP generates good feelings and helps us to create a more compelling future. As a therapist, it's a 'dream team' of a combination. Much more about NLP later, including techniques and guidelines to help *you* reprogramme your mind – once you have emptied your emotional barrel.

>>>Your 'Pain Body' – John's Story

I use the phrase 'Pain Body' to represent the pain in your body created by your mind. Most people know that amputees often suffer chronic pain where their amputated limb was; this confirms the belief that pain isn't always physically generated.

John was a client I worked with for a television series. He'd volunteered after Central ITV ran a campaign asking for people to write in and 'challenge' me to eliminate their problem using TFT. John was suffering from back pain and had been off work for some weeks and was considering surgery. He had been given the relevant medical checks by his doctor and the hospital and, although they acknowledged his pain and disability (he could barely get out of a chair), they could find no real cause for the extent of it, other than some not insignificant wear and tear on the spine.

A keen gardener, John was as eager to get back outside as he was to get back to work.

When I arrived, Alison, the reporter and presenter for the series, had set up the camera and was chatting to John, who could not even get up out of his chair to greet me. I chatted to John about his back pain (I have had a spinal fusion, so can empathize fully with the debilitating effects of back pain). John was pleased that I understood exactly what he was going through. We chatted about the fact that since my own surgery, which had been essential due to a series of small fractures in a vertebra in my lumbar spine, I was able to continue my then career as a personal trainer and aerobics instructor, and go on to train literally hundreds of other fitness instructors and open my own chain of health clubs, while teaching up to 11 fitness classes per week. Most other people I met in hospital having similar operations gave up exercise due to a 'bad back' and proceeded to gain weight, making the back problem worse … however, I will come back to mental attitude later!

There are some specific sequences, or algorithms, for pain, which I had planned to use with John and teach him to use himself. As is my normal pattern of working, especially when there is a chronic emotional or physical problem, I decided to check out John's 'emotional barrel'.

A quick chat revealed some pretty significant traumas from an early age. What they were was irrelevant, both for filming that day and for now; let's just call them 'the problems'. The significant point was that John's emotional barrel was full to bursting, even though he had 'no complaints' about his current life and had been 'happily settled' for some time. I asked him if he would mind me treating him for 'the problems' before we began treating his back pain. He agreed.

I asked him to tell me which events in his past had caused the most trauma and rate them on a scale of 1 to 10, with 10 being the worst. There were plenty of 10s on his list. This scale is called SUD, an abbreviation for Subjective Units of Distress. I will show you how to use this scale very soon. It is commonly used in various types of psychology, and is not exclusive to TFT.

Having identified the 'problems' that were the worst, I began to tap John. Within minutes he was visibly changing. He later described it as when birds tap their feet on the soil, using vibration to bring the worms to the top so they can be eaten. In John's words, 'I literally felt the emotion and its effects rise up and leave my body completely.' This is by no means a unique experience: some people feel 'it' go down and out through their feet, or even out through their chest, but a sense of feeling the 'problem' leave the body is very common. Often it elicits the response: 'That was weird!' In my work I have come to love the word 'weird', and now consider it a good sign when people say 'That was weird!'

After fewer than 15 minutes, John was visibly more relaxed and his posture had changed significantly. To assess how we were doing I asked him to get up out of the chair as if he were not in pain. He looked at me as if I were mad and then promptly stood up. I don't know who was more surprised, John or Alison, who suddenly shouted, 'No! He can't be fixed yet! We haven't filmed the "before" shots!' In the true spirit of television, John was promptly whisked outside and asked to pretend to try and dig the garden as if he were still in terrible pain, so the clip you can still see today on my website shows John's 'before' shot as if he is attempting to dig. In reality if we had filmed the 'before' shots before the treatment started, he wouldn't even have been able to hold the spade and stand upright.

We did not make the same mistake with any of the other volunteers for the programme, so when I worked with Kerry, our needle phobic, her extreme reaction to seeing a needle was filmed before the treatment and is in stark contrast to her holding a needle and lightly pricking her own skin fewer than 30 minutes later.

Meanwhile, back to John: I worked with him for another hour, after which we had cleared all the 'problems' and he could not recall the emotional pain he'd felt from any of the events. He was mystified. 'I don't know how it works ... but it works!' I hadn't even got as far as the specific treatment for pain, and yet all his pain had gone.

I saw John two weeks later for a follow-up appointment. He was able to drive to my house, some 60 minutes away, something he had been unable to do before the treatment. This in itself gave him back a significant level of independence. We cleared a few remaining minor issues that had surfaced since the original session, and used some NLP and hypnosis to generate lots of good feelings. As he was leaving, John said, 'By the way, since your treatment my psoriasis has started to clear up,' and proceeded to roll his trouser leg up and show me. I'd had no idea he had psoriasis, it wasn't *mentioned at our first meeting and I hadn't set out to clear it up – however, this kind of reaction is not uncommon with TFT. You'll be able appreciate why when you understand the physical connection between the emotional barrel and our Pain Body.*

The story doesn't end there – the following Christmas I had a lovely card from John, saying he had resigned his normal job and is now a full-time gardener. The following spring I received a beautiful hanging basket as a gift.

What to Tap and When

The tapping points we work with are located along specific meridian points. In TFT we use up to 14 treatment points, and 12 at algorithm level. For those of you interested in pure figures, Sean Quigley, one of only 12 certified TFT-VT practitioners, was intrigued as to how many possible combinations and different permutations could be diagnosed. He used the following formula to calculate this:

Allowing for the 12 relevant tapping points which can be repeated in a sequence if necessary (the precise order in which the points are tapped is significant), the formula is n to the power of r. This means that a potential 23,298,085,122,481 permutations are possible!

This demonstrates that random tapping is completely impractical. Imagine how many sequences you might have to try before you got the right combination?!

Through a diagnostic process, Dr Callahan identified a series of sequences that repeatedly showed up with clients with the same 'problem'. He realized that these sequences would eliminate the problem in approximately 80 per cent of cases. This level of TFT is known as *algorithm* level.

What Is an Algorithm?

An algorithm is of course not a new word, nor is it exclusive to TFT. Algorithm is a term used frequently in mathematics and in computer programming: to make a computer do what you want it to do, it has to have a programme or a set of instructions to follow, written in a specific language from which the computer can deduce its next move. In simple terms, it is a *formula*.

In reality, any set of instructions could be termed an algorithm – even taking a taxi ride:

- **Go to taxi rank.**
- **Get in taxi.**
- **Give your driver the address of your destination so he or she can take appropriate action.**
- **Pay the driver and get out of the taxi on arrival.**

A TFT algorithm, or *algo*, is used to describe a specific sequence of tapping points. This is the distinct difference between TFT and EFT. With EFT you tap all the treatment points in exactly the same order every time, while repeating statements out loud such as 'Even though I have this fear I totally and utterly accept myself.' Not everyone is comfortable doing this (I have used both methods and found this to be the case). With TFT it is not necessary to recite the problem out loud.

Imagine for a moment a Gatling gun. This is a machine gun that fires a large number of bullets at once at a given target. If you fire enough bullets, inevitably some will hit the target. Many of the bullets will miss, however, giving at best a partial result. Compare this to a laser-precision rifle, or a heat-seeking missile, that seeks out and finds the exact target and eliminates it.

Another example would be if you were to visit your GP with an infection and he or she gave you a broad-spectrum antibiotic known to kill several variations of bacteria.

There's a chance it may work, either completely or in part. Alternatively, if you had a blood test to identify the *specific* bacteria causing the illness, and your GP then prescribed the precise antibiotic, the bacteria would certainly be completely eliminated. In this same way, although EFT can be successful and is not to be dismissed, when compared to the precise way in which TFT works, EFT can be a much longer, less accurate process.

What Results Can You Expect to Achieve?

By following the step-by-step instructions carefully, you can replicate the success a TFT algorithm practitioner can achieve. In the next chapter, you will learn the 'protocol' for using TFT. As a result you will be able to treat and ultimately eliminate many negative emotions and problems such as anxiety, depression, phobias and many more.

Later in the book you will learn basic NLP techniques to complement TFT.

This is not a self-help book, it's a self-empowering book – and the power of these techniques is potentially ... life-changing.

Measuring Your Progress

Unlike clinical diagnostic techniques which can measure a biological response clinically, such as a blood test, psychological techniques are based on the individual's perception of the changes taking place. For this we use a scale called Subjective Units of Distress, or SUD for short. This scale is not exclusive to TFT. It is very useful. In practice it is quite simply a process of rating your 'problem' on a scale of 1–10, with 10 being the worst.

In order to get an accurate SUD reading, you must be in the *thought field*. This may mean taking a few minutes to remember *exactly* how you feel when you are in a given situation. For instance, if you are treating yourself for a past trauma, you need to re-access the memory of that event. That means being able to see what you saw, hear what you heard, and feel what you felt when the trauma occurred. Unlike counselling, you don't have to spend hours talking the episode through; you simply need to access the memory and its associated feelings for a few minutes so it can be eliminated.

If you are having trouble accessing the thought, there are some great resources you can use. One example is the YouTube website. I recently treated a woman for a butterfly phobia and she could not get in the 'thought field' just by thinking about it, but when I showed her a clip of butterflies on YouTube she got in the thought field straight away!

I have used the same technique for numerous phobics, including clips of fairground rides, spiders and flying.

If it is an emotion based around a person, looking at a picture of them, or even just writing down their name, can help access the thought.

Be aware that the SUD is not representing how you felt *at the time*, it represents how you feel when you re-access the thought and think about it *now*.

Golden rule number 1 in TFT: GET IN THE THOUGHT FIELD and then take an SUD reading.

When you have done this, rate it between 1 and 10, with 10 being the strongest and worst possible feeling, and 1 being that you can remember the event, but there's no emotion attached to it. Make a note of this number *before* you begin tapping. At each stage of the process you will be asked to take an SUD reading so that you can see how much of the problem each sequence has removed. This will tell you whether to repeat the same sequence or adapt it.

Using this system, there is no zero; 1 is the lowest possible score. The treatment is successful when the SUD is a 2 or 1. This means you can go on to the final stage of the treatment, which as you will see is called the 'eye roll'. If you are using TFT with children, then you can use a system of 'smiley/sad faces' if they cannot gauge a number accurately. Even some adults prefer this method! All you need is a diagram of a line of faces going from very sad to smiley. These can be very basic; simply a circle with eyes, a nose and a downward frown progressing gradually to a wide smile. Most charts go up in twos, so that would be five faces going from sad to happy.

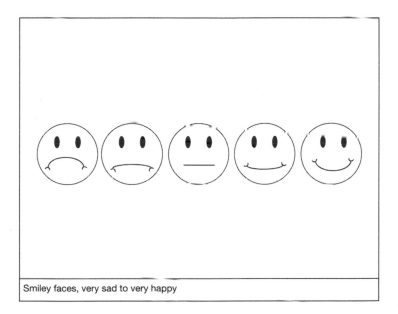

Smiley faces, very sad to very happy

One of the few factors that can block your success and prevent a reduction in your SUD is if you are in *Psychological Reversal* (PR). As mentioned earlier, this is when you are quite literally 'revorced' in the way you think and behave. We will cover this important aspect of TFT in more detail a bit later on, and you will see how easily it can be cleared, simply by tapping on the side of the hand as shown on page 7. And if that does not work, I will show you other corrective treatments later on that will allow the SUD to come down.

Knowing What to Treat

When I train therapists in TFT, apart from teaching them the correct protocol – that is, learning where the tapping points are and what algorithms to use – I emphasize how important it is to treat the correct emotion, which may not be the emotion that seemed uppermost at first. This, I believe, is the difference between being an average therapist and a *great* therapist. *You* can be the best possible therapist, even if you are only treating yourself, if you keep in mind what you are about to learn.

As mentioned earlier, if you want to use TFT to stop smoking or stop overeating, then it makes sense to eliminate the 'problems' or thoughts that cause you to smoke or overeat in the first place. If you are in the middle of a divorce, moving house, or in any stressful situation, it makes sense to eliminate that stress first before dealing with your cravings for tobacco or food.

Whatever you are using TFT for, please bear in mind the 'Barrel Effect' discussed earlier. Your life can be richly enhanced when you empty your emotional barrel. Even though the 'stuff' in there may not be related to the problems you may be experiencing now, lightening the emotional load makes a hugely significant difference.

When using TFT you may experience the 'peeling an onion' effect. This means that when you take away one 'layer' of the problem, another presents itself. This will be in the form of another thought around the same event. For example, follow the sequence of events below:

- A person is suffering from sadness as a result of a divorce/separation. This, like many other problems, is a multilayered emotional trauma. The following list is hypothetical but gives you an idea of the onion effect.
- Initial algorithm (*algo*) is used to gauge the trauma of the event.
- The trauma is eliminated and now the feeling is anger.
- *Algo* is used to eliminate the anger.
- The anger is eliminated and now there is sadness.
- *Algo* is used to eliminate the sadness.
- The sadness is eliminated and now there's fear about facing the future alone.
- Anxiety/fear *algo* (*see* page 176) is used.
- Anxiety and fear removed; now there's lack of confidence.
- *Algo* used for self-esteem and confidence.

As you can see, once one 'layer' of a problem is eliminated, another appears.

If you are not treating a trauma but are treating a phobia, of flying for example, the fears to address may proceed like this:

- anxiety the night before the flight, worrying about it
- the check-in process – all the security measures, etc.
- boarding the plane
- take-off
- feeling closed in once the plane is airborne
- turbulence
- landing.

If you are treating for a fear of spiders or any other animal, treatment might proceed like this:

- **getting used to a picture of a spider**
- **seeing a real-life spider**
- **seeing a spider move**
- **getting used to spiders with large bodies**
- **getting used to spiders with long legs**
- **overcoming fear of a picture of a tarantula**
- **picking up or removing a spider.**

As you can see, there are many layers to any given problem. Sometimes, however, you can clear several levels all at once! But be ready to be patient and systematic in your treatment if you need to.

Often when I am working with clients for weight loss, it becomes apparent that their self-esteem is very low, which is usually a result of some past experiences. Once these issues are cleared, then the cause of the 'problem' is cleared. A side effect of TFT is that you just might start feeling good … for no reason whatsoever!

Start at the Beginning

Another technique I teach all my students is to *start at the beginning*. By this I mean that if you are treating someone for blushing, for example, GO BACK to the beginning and find the time when the blushing first began.

A very common fear or phobia is of public speaking; clearing the anxiety is much easier once you remove the cause. Go back and remember the time you had your first ever or worst ever experience in front of people, and clear that before you clear the anxiety you have now.

>>>Dave's Story

Dave came to see me for a fear of public speaking, which is one of the most common phobias. As usual I asked him to tell me when the phobia began, or what might have triggered it. He could not recall any event that might explain this fear. It came about whenever he had to make a presentation at work, and as he had climbed the ladder within his company this was becoming more and more necessary. These presentations usually related to projects involving sums of money in excess of several million pounds. It would be normal for most of us in these circumstances to feel some pressure, some desire to want to get it right. A certain amount of pressure can actually be helpful – ask any athlete if they would like to compete in an Olympic final without producing adrenaline and they would soon tell you 'NO!' – but too much and our imagination runs wild and it becomes counterproductive.

A phobia is when the normal level of fear is surpassed and, in a completely irrational way, increased to often extreme levels. I explained to Dave that this kind of phobia is a learned behaviour, not something you are born with, and that somewhere in his past he either experienced or witnessed an event that triggered this irrational fear. I asked him if he had ever been embarrassed at school, perhaps in a school play or assembly. He immediately remembered that as a teenager they were all asked to stand up and chat for a minute about what they wanted to do for a job when they left school. Dave stood up and proudly spoke of his desire to be in the RAF. When he had finished his teacher said, 'Well, that's OK if you want to kill people.' There was a stunned silence in the room and everyone looked at Dave, who was absolutely mortified and sat down, quite unable to speak or respond. Later on when his parents found out, they went into the school and the teacher was 'spoken to' and apologies made, but the damage had been done. This experience had given Dave a very good reason not to want to stand up and speak in front of a group.

I treated Dave by first using the trauma sequence I will show you later in the book. We treated it from every angle. He remembered how sick he felt 'in the pit of his stomach', so he held that thought while we tapped. Then we used the trauma with anger sequence (page 191) while he was thinking specifically about the teacher, then the trauma with embarrassment sequence (page 191) as he thought about how he'd felt as he stood there. Each was an individual layer of the same event or problem, and by eliminating all the layers we completely cleared any negative effects of the event. We then treated more recent events, from meetings at work to interviews, in a similar way; all were successfully diminished with TFT. Then I asked him to 'future pace' and imagine he had a meeting in 5 minutes, and to get as anxious as he could. Thinking about this prospect, he was around a 5 on the SUD scale. So we tapped for that, and after a few minutes he could not re-experience the anxious feeling at all.

Since the treatment, Dave has gone from strength to strength and public speaking is no longer the daunting prospect it once was. While we could have just addressed the immediate fear of speaking in public, by being thorough and clearing all the layers, Dave got the best possible result and is now free to achieve his full potential, at work and in all areas of his life.

Why TFT May Not Work

The average success rate for TFT is between 70 and 85 per cent when the techniques are applied correctly. As with any method, the more accomplished you become, the better the results you can achieve. Ask any medical practitioner: if they could prescribe a drug or a treatment which had an up to 85 per cent success rate, they would probably bite your hand off to get it! These kinds of results are unprecedented in therapy.

As good as it is, however, TFT does not work for everyone. Dr Callahan himself has a phrase for this: 'Anyone who says they have a 100 per cent success rate hasn't treated enough people yet!' The good news is that we know the reasons why TFT may not work, and most are preventable:

- **The person is not in the Thought Field (TF).**
- **The person is using the wrong sequence (algorithm).**
- **The person is in Psychological Reversal (PR).**
- **The person has Individual Energy Toxins (IETs) present.**

The most common of these, assuming the treatment is being carried out correctly, is Psychological Reversal (PR). (For more about PR, see the next chapter.)

Negative Polarity

The term 'polarity' relates to a basic law of nature: electro-magnetic force, or attraction and repulsion. It centres around the attraction and union of opposites through a balanced middle point. The human body is effectively an electrical plant, running on high-voltage energy. If there's a short in the circuits, or an injury to the system, the circuit breakers can shut the whole system down. This is effectively what happens when we are in PR.

To maintain optimal health, life energy must be able to flow freely throughout the body.

As mentioned earlier in the book, correcting PR is, in his own words, Dr Callahan's most important discovery.

He is not the only person to have investigated the dramatic effects of reversed polarity in the body: the Austrian-American chiropractor, osteopath and naturopath Randolph Stone (1888–1981) dedicated much of his life and work to this endeavour, and went on to develop Polarity Therapy as an integration of Eastern and Western principles and techniques of healing. Others who have worked in this area and achieved favourable results in maintaining a positive polarity in terms of health and healing include Harold Saxton Burr (1889–1973), a biology professor at Yale who believed that all living things possessed electro-magnetic polarity. He used a simple voltmeter to demonstrate this. I will show you how to replicate this later in this book.

In 1972 Louis Langham, a medical professor of gynaecology, showed that most patients who had malignant tumours showed a negative polarity when compared to non-malignant subjects, who showed a mostly positive polarity. In tests Professor Langham found that 96 per cent of patients with malignancy showed a negative polarity, whereas 95 per cent of his cancer-free subjects showed a positive polarity.

You can access this study in an article by Joanne Callahan at www.rogercallahan.com/cancer.php

Others who have examined the energy forces and polarity of the body and the negative effects on our health include James Oschman, PhD, in *Energy Medicine* and Dr Andrew Weil in his book, *Spontaneous Healing*. Most Polarity Therapy practitioners use various forms of physical manipulation and pressure to release blocked energy, often along the meridian lines, together with prescribing exercise (such as yoga) and nutritional advice.

Where Dr Callahan had been visionary was in his discovery that simply by tapping certain key points on the body you can, in most cases, clear a negative polarity, making TFT a uniquely straightforward and effective treatment which can, in most cases, have amazing psychological and physiological benefits.

Psychological Reversal: When Your Mind Does the Opposite of What You Want It To

The effects of being in PR are far-reaching, both emotionally and physically. When you are 'reversed' you may experience the following symptoms:

- **constant negativity**
- **procrastination**
- **self-sabotaging behaviour**
- **reversing words or actions, for example turning left when you know you should be turning right, putting the dinner in the fridge and the milk in the oven**
- **dyslexia or other problems processing information**
- **generally feeling in a muddle and not understanding things**
- **failure to heal physically.**

There are two classifications of PR:

1. **MASSIVE REVERSAL**
2. **SPECIFIC REVERSAL.**

Let's deal with the emotional effects first. If you read the above list and can relate to some or all of the above being present in your life on a regular basis, then the chances are you are in MASSIVE REVERSAL. This means that for no apparent reason whatsoever, you are constantly experiencing some form of negativity or lack of understanding. No matter what you are thinking about, you are in MASSIVE PR.

If you feel OK most of the time but experience some of the symptoms mentioned at certain times, say for example if you are learning to speak French and yet when you look at or hear the words your brain does not process the information and it gets all muddled, causing you confusion and frustration, then this is a SPECIFIC PR. That is, you are reversed to learning French. When you think about anything else you feel positive, but when you think about learning French, you get in a muddle.

In terms of health, if you show a negative reading on a voltmeter (more on this in a moment), this indicates MASSIVE REVERSAL.

There are a few ways you can check for reversal, other than just by experiencing the symptoms and noting them. One is with a voltmeter.

Testing for PR using a Voltmeter

You should find detailed directions and diagrams in the instructions for your voltmeter, but here are the basic guidelines:

- **Using a highly sensitive digital voltmeter, hold the black point in your left hand with your left thumb lightly on the point.**
- **Hold the red lead in your right hand and place the point gently on the back of your left hand.**
- **Take the reading.**

- **The reading on the screen of the voltmeter will give you a number; If it is positive then you are NOT in PR. If, however, it is negative, you ARE in PR and should follow the corrective sequence shown at the end of this chapter (page 60).**

It is also possiblo to have a SPECIFIC *PHYSICAL* REVERSAL. In this instance you would have a positive reading when using a voltmeter, but then if you were to place the point of the red lead directly on, say, the site of an injury (rather than on the back of your left hand) you would get a negative reading. This would be termed a SPECIFIC REVERSAL for that precise physical location.

An example of this from my own life is that in 2006 I underwent a minor gynaecological procedure which involved a small incision just below my belly button. The scar was no more than 2 cm long. I was quite poorly after the operation, which was largely investigative in nature, and had to stay overnight instead of being released at 5 p.m. on the same day as predicted. The next morning I went home, still feeling very sore around the wound. Aftor a few days it just was not healing and looked no different to the day after surgery. I decided to test myself by placing the voltmeter on my hand. It measured positive. But when I placed it on the injury site, it plummeted to a reading of -200. I then placed my hand over the wound and began to tap my PR spot while my hand covered the wound. I did this several times an hour. When I checked later in the day, the polarity had leapt up to +50, and almost before my eyes the wound began to heal. I continued to tap and within 24 hours there was a thin scab, and within a few days the wound had healed completely.

Last year I developed, almost overnight, a large abscess inside my gum above my teeth. I went to see my dentist, who X-rayed it and told me it would require surgery and a general anaesthetic. He said he was going to have to drill a hole in the bone and drain the infection, as it had probably been there for years. I left the surgery and once again placed my hand over the injury site and tapped the PR spot on it. I did this many times a day over the next fortnight. When I went back two weeks later the abscess had shrunk by over 50 per cent. My dentist, however, was unimpressed, and insisted I go to the hospital to see the maxillofacial consultant. By the time the appointment came through several months later, and with repeated tapping on the PR spot while my hand was over my mouth, there was no visible sign of the abscess. As my dentist had told me that the worst of the infection was inside the bone, however, I went along for the appointment none the less. When I arrived they X-rayed me and, after a very long wait, the consultant came out and said to me, 'Apologies for the delay; we have been checking with your dentist as to why he referred you, as we can find nothing wrong!' All signs of the abscess, both externally and inside the bone, had vanished.

> *It's important to emphasize here that tapping the PR spot does not 'heal' you. What it does is prevent the negative polarity from blocking the body's natural healing process. If you stay positive your body is more able to perform its natural ability to repair itself.*

In reality, we are all in and out of reversal all the time. Exercise can clear a reversal, for example, which is why sometimes after a good workout things don't seem so bad! Sean Quigley and I ran some experiments in which we bounced on a rebounder whenever we felt reversed and tested negative, and we found that after two minutes of bouncing, the reversal almost always cleared. It was interesting, but of course not as quick and easy as tapping the side of your hand for 20 seconds!

I smile now as I write this, because when I got to the part about rebounders, I could not remember the correct name for them. I was getting frustrated, and about to type in 'mini-trampoline'; however, when tapping the side of my hand the word 'rebounder' popped back into my head. A case in point, I think! I have used this simple technique many times when I can't remember where I've put something; as if by magic, after tapping I always remember just where it is.

Arm Testing for PR

As mentioned, there are a few ways you can check for reversal; with a voltmeter, as discussed, and with the help of a friend, using the basic form of muscle testing commonly used in applied kinesiology.

Applied kinesiology is a therapy based on muscle testing, which you can use literally to 'ask your body' questions and get an accurate non-verbal answer. This technique involves two people. The most important element is learning to *calibrate* first.

Stand with feet hip-width apart, and raise one arm out to the side. Have your partner press down firmly on your arm and you resist the pressure so that your arm stays strong and does not lower under the pressure. You BOTH need to

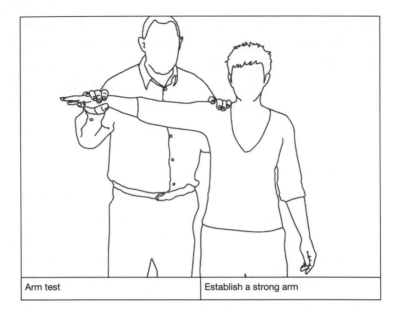

Arm test	Establish a strong arm

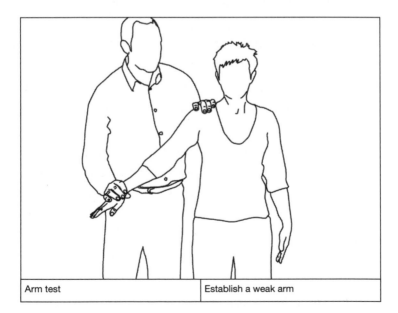

Arm test	Establish a weak arm

calibrate how firm your actions are. The aim is to find out how much pressure you need to exert to keep your arm strong; it's not about who is the strongest. Clearly the amount of pressure the tester exerts on your arm will vary according to how strong each of you is.

Once you have calibrated, move on to the next phase, which is to test for Psychological Reversal: stand upright and place your left arm over your head (but not touching it), palm facing downwards. Have your partner press firmly down on your right arm as you resist, holding your arm still.

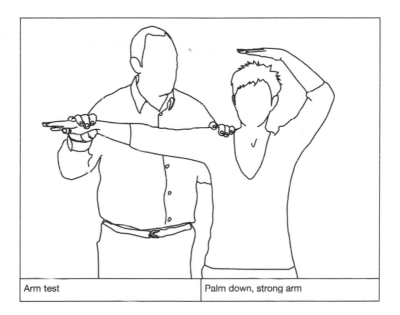

| Arm test | Palm down, strong arm |

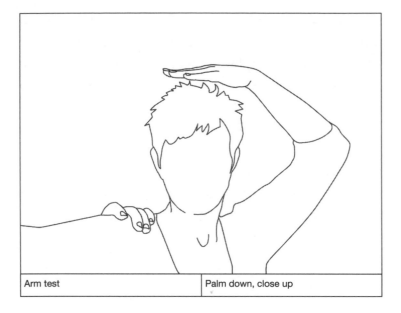

Arm test	Palm down, close up

Notice how strong you feel and the exact amount of effort it takes you to resist. You need to assess just how much pressure you both need to exert for your arm to stay in the same position. If your partner is much stronger than you, do not allow them to press so hard your arm collapses. Between the two of you, work out how hard you have to resist to keep your right arm in the same position, and how much pressure the other person can exert until just before your arm drops. It is important your partner exerts a constant pressure, for about 3–4 seconds. They press, you resist.

Now turn your left hand so the back of your hand is facing your head and the palm is facing up. Have your partner exert the same amount of pressure as before and resist.

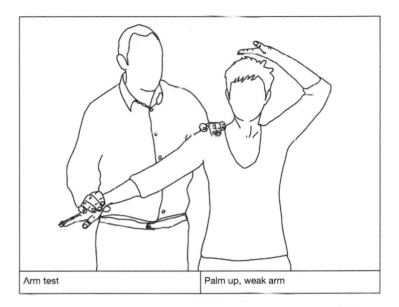

| Arm test | Palm up, weak arm |

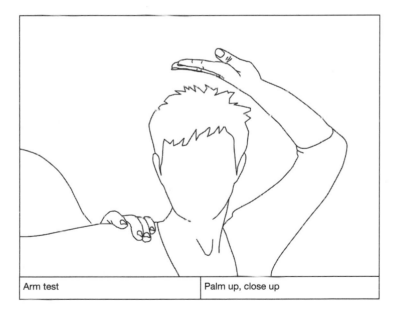

| Arm test | Palm up, close up |

You will probably notice a drastic difference between the two, in that with your palm facing down, your arm is strong, as this has positive polarity, and when you flip over so the palm is facing up, your arm is weak, as this has negative polarity.

If you are NOT in reversal you will find that
PALM DOWN = STRONG/POSITIVE
PALM UP = WEAK/NEGATIVE

If both are the same strength, or the results are the wrong way round – i.e. palm down = weak, palm up = strong, it indicates a MASSIVE REVERSAL. You need to use the corrective treatments shown at the end of this chapter.

Alternatively, instead of using the palm up/palm down method, place one arm out to the side (keep the other one beside your body) and have your partner apply steady pressure for 3–4 seconds. Say 'My name is ...' (saying your correct name) as you resist and notice how strong your arm is. Rest for a few seconds and then repeat, but this time say 'My name is Daffy Duck' and, with your partner exerting the same pressure, notice how weak your arm becomes in comparison to when you are telling the truth.

This technique is reliable for almost everyone. Occasionally someone cannot feel a difference, and this indicates the presence of toxins. This toxicity problem will be discussed later in the book, and can be identified and corrected using TFT Voice Technology (*see* page 100).

Sometimes if there is a drastic physical difference between tester and testee, then it can be difficult to feel the difference, but in most cases this is a practical and reliable method that can be used effectively by most people.

Once you have identified a clear difference, so that palm down – strong and palm up = weak, you can use muscle testing to ask your body and your unconscious mind questions. In simple terms, a strong arm = YES and a weak arm = NO.

We learned earlier that what we think can affect us physically by filling up our 'emotional barrel'. If you want to test for yourself how much a negative thought can affect you physically, try this:

Think about someone or something that makes you feel good. Something or someone special that makes you feel empowered. Hold that thought NOW and really focus on it. When you have got the thought, raise your arm to the side and have your partner press down while you resist the pressure. If you are not reversed, your arm will be STRONG while you have this thought.

Now think about someone or somewhere you don't like. Hold that thought for a moment and focus on it and, while you hold the thought, repeat the arm test. Your arm will probably be weak; that means that when you think about this event or this person you are not only emotionally weakened, but physically weakened as well.

If you have identified a thought or memory that makes your arm weak, this needs removing using the corrective treatment shown at the end of this chapter. In addition you may require one of the appropriate algorithms shown in later chapters. The thought or memory is literally weakening you physically and emotionally.

If your arm is strong on both counts, you are in PR. This can also be corrected (see page 60) and you can then re-do the exercise.

Corrective Treatment

There are several elements to correcting PR. In most cases, Stages 1 and 3 are sufficient.

In all cases if you are using corrective treatment because TFT is not working, then it is important to remain focused on the problem while using the treatment.

• **Tap the side of your hand 20+ times (karate spot). This is known as PR1.**

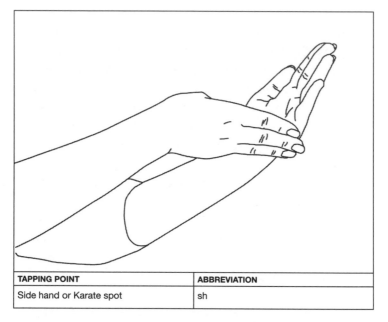

TAPPING POINT	ABBREVIATION
Side hand or Karate spot	sh

• **Run your fingers along the underside of your LEFT collarbone from the shoulder to the centre of your chest. If you find a spot that is sore, then gently but firmly rub this spot using circular motions towards the centre of your chest, until the soreness subsides. If you do have a sore spot (and you may not) this indicates the possible presence** of toxins in your body, as this is where the lymphatic system meets the blood circulation. This may require further investigation and is discussed in more detail later on.

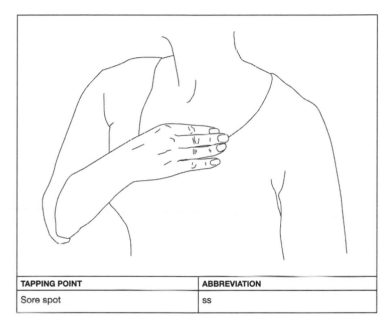

TAPPING POINT	ABBREVIATION
Sore spot	SS

- Tap under your nose 20+ times. This is known as PR2.

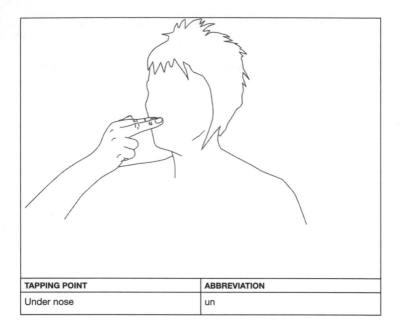

TAPPING POINT	ABBREVIATION
Under nose	un

• **Do collarbone breathing.**

Collarbone Breathing (cb2)

If tapping the side of your hand (indicated in TFT with the initials **sh**) to correct PR is likened to clicking 'refresh page' on your computer while surfing the Internet, then cb2 can be likened to a complete reboot of the system.

While tapping **sh** should be done regularly throughout the day, cb2 should be done morning and evening for most people. Those with ongoing anxiety, chronic addictions or OCD will benefit from doing cb2 at least three times a day. It uses the tapping of meridian points combined with the body's natural polarity in order to achieve balance. It is generally only used as part of a treatment if an *algo* is not working and the SUD is not coming down.

Note: The back of the hand has a different polarity to the palm of the hand; this is the reason we fold the fingers under and use the knuckles for certain positions. It is important to prevent the thumb or the elbows from touching the body at any time, as this can 'short' the circuit.

1. **Place two fingers of one hand (positive polarity) on one collarbone (keep thumb clear).**
2. **Using the other hand, tap the gamut spot (on the back of your hand between the little finger and ring finger knuckles) continuously while doing the following breathing technique:**

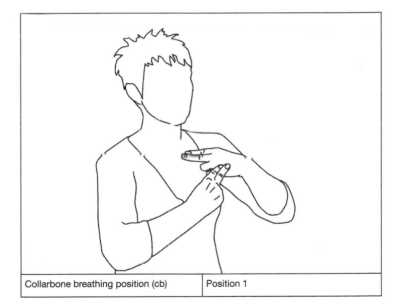

Collarbone breathing position (cb)	Position 1

- **Breathe all the way in and hold for a few seconds.**
- **Let half the breath out and hold.**
- **Let all the breath out and hold.**

- Breathe half the way in and hold.
- Breathe out.

3. Move the fingers across to the other collarbone and repeat the process.
4. Now curl the fingers underneath (tuck the thumb inside or keep clear) and place the knuckles (negative polarity) onto the collarbone, tap the gamut spot continuously and repeat the breathing sequence (see illustration below).

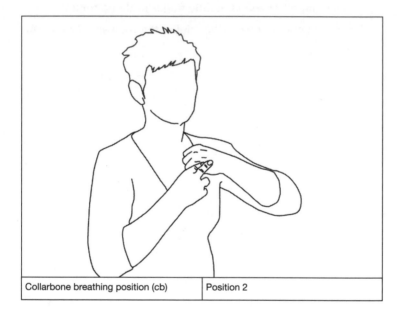

| Collarbone breathing position (cb) | Position 2 |

5. Move your fist across to the other collarbone and repeat the process.
6. Change hands and repeat the tapping and breathing with the fingers on each collarbone, then repeat with knuckles.

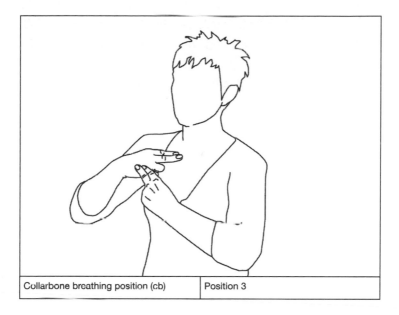

| Collarbone breathing position (cb) | Position 3 |

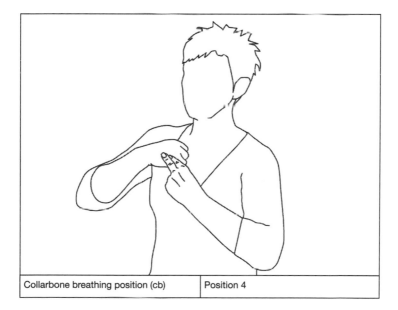

| Collarbone breathing position (cb) | Position 4 |

You have completed the exercise when you have done both positions (i.e. fingers and knuckles) on both collarbones with both hands.

Part 2
Practising TFT

Tapping Points

Now it's time to learn about the specific TFT points in more detail, where they are and what they represent, before we put it all together and learn how to apply TFT in a simple, effective way.

Important Note: it does NOT matter which side of the body you tap.

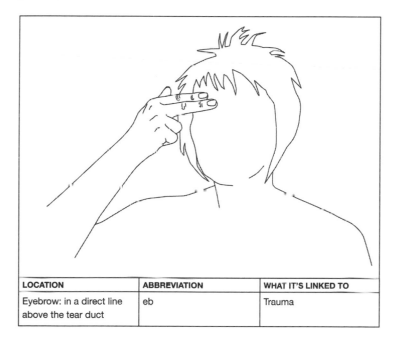

LOCATION	ABBREVIATION	WHAT IT'S LINKED TO
Eyebrow: in a direct line above the tear duct	eb	Trauma

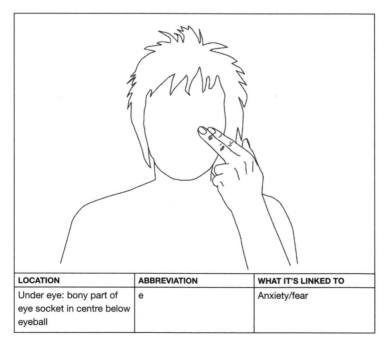

LOCATION	ABBREVIATION	WHAT IT'S LINKED TO
Outside eye: on temple	oe	Rage

LOCATION	ABBREVIATION	WHAT IT'S LINKED TO
Under eye: bony part of eye socket in centre below eyeball	e	Anxiety/fear

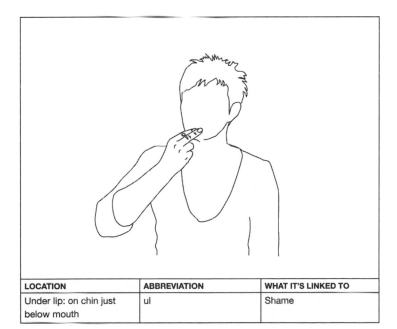

LOCATION	ABBREVIATION	WHAT IT'S LINKED TO
Under nose: between nose and lip	un	Embarrassment and PR2

LOCATION	ABBREVIATION	WHAT IT'S LINKED TO
Under lip: on chin just below mouth	ul	Shame

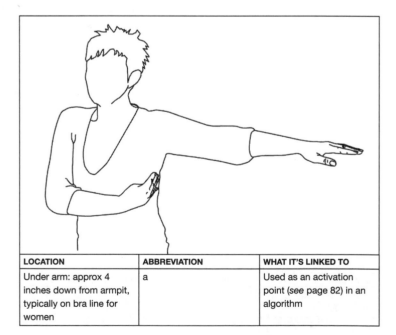

LOCATION	ABBREVIATION	WHAT IT'S USED FOR
Collarbone: at base of throat, feel for the notch in the bone and move 1 inch along bone away from centre, and 1 inch down	c	Punctuation in an algorithm and for cb2

LOCATION	ABBREVIATION	WHAT IT'S LINKED TO
Under arm: approx 4 inches down from armpit, typically on bra line for women	a	Used as an activation point (see page 82) in an algorithm

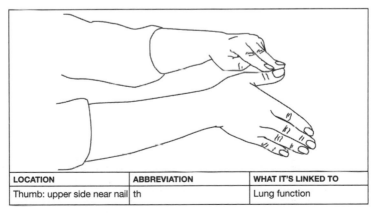

LOCATION	ABBREVIATION	WHAT IT'S LINKED TO
Sore spot – run fingers along the underside (between 1 and 3 inches below) of LEFT collarbone between shoulder and chest. (You may not have one; this is fine.)	ss	The presence of toxins and/or reversals

Important Note: For ALL finger positions, hold the hand out as if to shake someone else's hand, with the thumb pointing UP. ALL finger points are tapped on the upper side with the hand in this position. It does NOT matter which hand you use.

LOCATION	ABBREVIATION	WHAT IT'S LINKED TO
Thumb: upper side near nail	th	Lung function

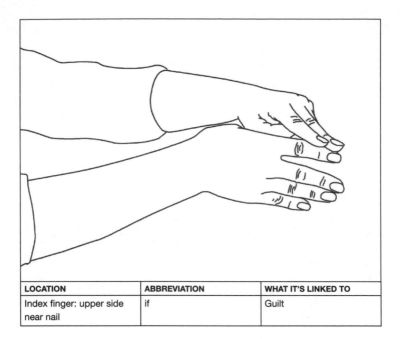

LOCATION	ABBREVIATION	WHAT IT'S LINKED TO
Index finger: upper side near nail	if	Guilt

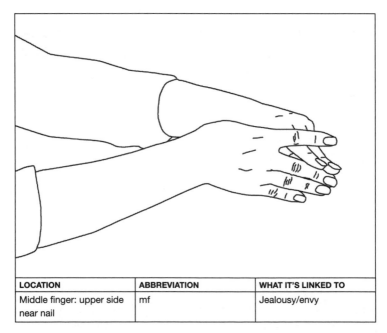

LOCATION	ABBREVIATION	WHAT IT'S LINKED TO
Middle finger: upper side near nail	mf	Jealousy/envy

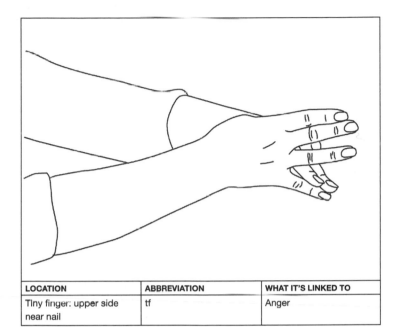

LOCATION	ABBREVIATION	WHAT IT'S LINKED TO
TIny finger: upper side near nail	tf	Anger

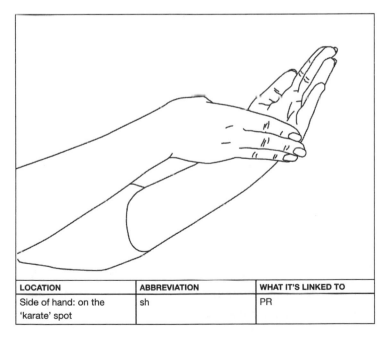

LOCATION	ABBREVIATION	WHAT IT'S LINKED TO
Side of hand: on the 'karate' spot	sh	PR

LOCATION	ABBREVIATION	WHAT IT'S LINKED TO
Gamut spot: on back of hand between tiny finger and ring finger knuckles	g (as 9g or g50)	Sadness/pain

All of these meridian points were identified by Dr Callahan as significant in the treatment of emotional and other psychological disturbances. It is the order and sequence of the points used that makes TFT so effective. It really is as simple as it is brilliant.

The sore spot (ss) is not technically a tapping point, and does not appear in the sequences you will learn, but it can be used to remove blockages if a treatment is not working. It is the point where the lymphatic system meets the blood's circulation system; if it is sore it can indicate the presence of toxins, which can block treatment. Once you have checked for a sore spot and failed to find one, there's no need to check at every stage of treatment. If there is one there, simply rub it gently until it has diminished.

The last spot listed above is the *gamut* spot, mentioned earlier. This treatment point forms the basis of a short sub-sequence (9g) used within every treatment. The purpose is to use movements and vocalizations that require both the right brain and the left brain to function while continually tapping the gamut spot. Read through the directions, then actually try out the 9g so you get used to doing it. As it features in every treatment, it is helpful to learn it off by heart. It is named 9g as there are nine components to it.

While continually tapping the gamut spot:

1. **Close your eyes (long blink).**
2. **Open your eyes.**
3. **Keeping your head still and moving your eyes only, look down to one side (R) and back to centre.**
4. **Look down to the other (L) side and back to centre.**
5. **Look down as if you were looking at number 6 on a clock dial, then move your eyes up and round in a circle as if you are looking at every number on the dial, finishing back at number 6.**
6. **Now repeat the circle but in the other direction.**
7. **Hum a few notes (e.g. the musical scales or 'happy birthday') out loud.**
8. **Count out loud 1-2-3-4-5.**
9. **Hum out loud again (the vibration of the hum is vital; make sure you hum, not sing).**

There is one other process that features at the end of every successful treatment, assuming the SUD (Subjective Units of

Distress) reading has reduced to a 2 or a 1. This is known as the *eye roll*. Think of this as clicking 'Save' on your computer.

The Eye Roll

Try this now: tap the gamut spot continuously and, keeping your head still, look directly downwards to your chest, then, as you continue to tap, slowly roll your eyes upwards until you are looking up at your eyebrows or as far as you can. This process should be done slowly and take about 10 seconds.

Protocol

Whichever sequence or *algo* you use, there is a certain protocol to follow:

1. Identify the problem.
2. Tune in to the thought field.
3. Take an SUD reading (1–10).
4. Select the correct *algo*.
5. Begin sequence/*algo*, tapping each point at least 15 times firmly but not too hard.
6. Take an SUD reading; if it has gone down 2 points or more, continue to next phase (7); if not, read more about corrective treatments (covered in the next chapter).
7. Do the 9 gamut (9g) sequence.
8. Repeat the sequence/*algo*.
9. Take an SUD reading. If it has gone down to a 2 or 1, do the eye roll; if it is still above a 2, then repeat the procedure (steps 1–9).

If after the first sequence there is no change in your SUD, then it is likely to be because of one of four things:

1. **You are not in the thought field.**
2. **You are using the wrong algo (sequence).**
3. **You are in PR.**
4. **There are IETs (toxins) present (more about this in a later chapter).**

Corrective Treatments

Assuming you are tuned in to the thought field and you have chosen the correct sequence for your particular problem, you can usually clear any reversals as follows:

- **Tap the side of the hand on the 'karate' spot (sh).**
- **Rub sore spot (ss) – if there is one.**
- **Tap under nose (un).**

This process alone may reduce the SUD, but even if it does not, repeat the tapping sequence for your particular problem. If the SUD has now started to reduce by more than 1 point, continue the protocol as described on page 78 from (7).

If repeating the protocol does not reduce the problem, having cleared PR, do cb2 (*see* page 62) while staying in the thought field, and begin again. If this has not reduced the SUD there is no point in repeating the process, as there is something else blocking treatment.

Bear in mind that in 70–80 per cent of cases, if you have followed the protocol correctly, you will get a good result. It is in the minority of cases that other factors block treatment.

Now you have read the basic protocol, it's time to have a go. There are chapters later in the book for specific problems and conditions, but for now, and so you can experience TFT at a basic level, just think about something that makes you anxious. Really focus on it and get tuned in to the thought. If it's a fear or a phobia, imagine you are in that situation now.

Take a few minutes to do so. Take an SUD reading and write it down.

Now tap the following sequence while focusing on the problem:

- **Under eye (e)**
- **Under arm (a)**
- **Collarbone (c).**

Take an SUD; if it has gone down 2 or more points, continue to the next phase. If not, tap side hand (**sh**), check for a sore spot (**ss**) and tap under the nose (**un**), then repeat the sequence.

If there is still no reduction in SUD of 2 or more, do cb2 while thinking of the anxiety.

- **Repeat the sequence.**
- **9g.**
- **Take an SUD.**

In most cases you will experience a reduction in the strength of the negative emotion. You simply repeat the whole cycle until the SUD is a 2 or 1, and then do the eye roll.

As mentioned in earlier chapters, some cases can be multilayered and complex. For now, just practise the basic technique and get used to the terms, doing the **9g** and the eye roll to familiarize yourself with the process. You also need to practise the cb2 procedure shown on page 62. That means put the book down and do both cb2 and **9g** now!

Welcome Back

Now you have had a chance to experience the process of TFT, you can begin to understand its elegance and simplicity. In fact it's so simple that often when I have eliminated a problem for someone, they cannot attribute the success to the simple process of tapping. How can it be that a problem they have had for years is gone in just a few minutes? They then decide that they can't remember the fear because 'the tapping distracts me'. This is called the Apex problem; in short, it's when people fail to accept that TFT has eliminated the problem.

>>>Tina's Story

One afternoon I was working from home catching up on admin, when I had a very distressing enquiry from a young woman of 21. Although I had promised myself an admin day, she was so upset I arranged to see her that afternoon for an emergency appointment. She was suffering from unexplained anxiety, almost 24/7. When she arrived she was very tearful and physically in a bad way, shaking and rocking. I chatted to her about what she wanted from the session (although it was obvious, it's important for individuals to focus on what they want to achieve, as it aids treatment). She said she wanted to stop feeling anxious about her future and stop drinking so much. I asked her a few questions, starting with 'What's the worst thing that has ever happened to you?' at which point she recalled a traumatic event with her mother and brother that resulted in a family split. As is often the case with this kind of event, there were many layers to this which we worked through for about 90 minutes. After this she just could not get any of the anxiety back; even though I asked her to try and get the negative feelings back, she could not. As she left she booked another session for the following week, as I felt that some NLP and perhaps hypnosis would give her a much more positive outlook on her future now the negativity had gone. When the appointment time arrived she did not turn up. I rang her to see if she was running late and she told me, 'I don't think the TFT worked for me; on the way home I gave myself a really good talking to and after that I felt much better. I have hardly had a drink since.' She had deleted the fact that she had been giving herself a good talking to for seven years without any effect at all, other than to make it worse!

This is a classic example of the Apex problem. As a therapist it can be frustrating, but on the basis that I do this job because I love helping people, as long as she is fixed then I have achieved my goal. For those clients who do attribute their success to the treatment, well, that's the icing on the cake for me.

TFT and the Medical Profession

There are, thank goodness, general practitioners, consultants and other medical professionals who now recognize the importance of integrating complementary therapies with traditional medicine. It is unfortunate that many clinicians dismiss such therapies out of hand due to lack of academic support or research. While it's true that there are some whacky theories out there, it's vital we do not throw the baby out with the bathwater. Dr Callahan himself struggled (and still does, within some academic fields) to have his discoveries acknowledged and credited. The good news, however, is that more and more medical practitioners are now recognizing and recommending drug-free psychological techniques, of which TFT is paramount in its success rate.

One of these forward-thinking and open-minded practitioners is Dr Mark Chambers, who has been working as a GP for 27 years and is actively involved in training other GPs; Dr Chambers has trained in TFT and now uses it regularly with patients in his practice. I have been lucky enough to work with Mark on a number of occasions, and have asked him to share with you directly his thoughts as a medical practitioner, in his own words:

>>>Thought Field Therapy in General Practice
I have been a general practitioner for 27 years. It is a challenging and stimulating calling, and I love it. The complexity of modern life brings a wide range of

problems to the GP's consulting room, far beyond the scope of what might be termed conventional medicine. In a recent census, when asked to give a brief description of his job, one GP replied: 'Anything, for anybody, anytime, anywhere'. One of the many privileges a GP enjoys is that, once the strictly medical aspects of a situation are addressed, he or she gets to choose how much further to go in helping the patient in front of him or her.

Modern Western medicine has evolved to a place now where there are very effective treatments for many conditions for which, only a generation or so ago, there was very little that could be done. The pharmaceutical industry continues to invest heavily in research and development, and new drugs are emerging all the time that expand the options of the medical profession for dealing with illness and disease. Similar progress is being made in surgical technology and technique. This is paralleled in psychological medicine, where new approaches and techniques are being researched and implemented all the time.

Despite all the above progress, there are still aspects of people's problems for which conventional medicine has, at best, a limited response. Happily, the same evolutionary process as outlined above has been taking place in many fields of complementary therapy.

This has often been led by conventionally-trained doctors and therapists who have become frustrated by the limitations of their conventional training when it comes to helping some of their patients and their particular problems effectively. Many new lines of therapy are emerging that are proving to be very effective and useful additions to the therapeutic tool kit. Thought Field Therapy is one of these.

My first introduction to Thought Field Therapy came a few years ago, when it was introduced during some advanced communication skills training I was taking, as part of my own personal development as a GP trainer. I was immediately impressed by its simplicity and how quick, simple and effective some TFT interventions can be. These properties make TFT particularly applicable to the time available in a typical GP consultation.

In general practice, as in much of modern life, time is the scarcest resource. We have, on average, 10 minutes with each patient at a time. In this time, research has demonstrated an average of three problems will emerge which require attention. Our conventional training has equipped us with the skills to address whatever arises in the course of a consultation, although our ability to intervene effectively varies according to the condition we are faced with. In the British National Health Service, the GP is essentially the gatekeeper of the service. He or she is usually the first port of call for the patient with a problem, and 19 out of 20 problems are dealt with within general practice. One in 20 problems is referred on to another part of the health or community services for further intervention.

This system works very well most of the time, but there are occasions where matters have come to a standstill but onward referral is not an option. Sometimes the necessary services are not available, or waiting times are long. Sometimes the patient does not wish to be referred on. In these situations it is very helpful, as a GP, to have some extra resources to offer. Equally,

*many patients have concerns about such issues as
the safety of modern conventional interventions, or
reservations about how some medicines are developed
and prepared. These patients often take an interest in
complementary approaches, and will often seek out a
GP sympathetic to their views.*

*Thought Field Therapy is an intervention which is ideally
suited to fill many of these gaps. As well as addressing
psychological and emotional issues, TFT can be applied
to many aspects of physical illness to good effect. It has
the virtue that, in many cases, it is very quick to apply,
and thus lends itself well to the 10-minute consultations
we work with. Most problems can be treated with
simple TFT techniques which are straightforward and
easy to learn, and quickly become very efficient with
practice. There are simple TFT interventions which
I regularly use for such problems as anxiety states,
phobias, weight loss, smoking cessation, compulsive
behaviours and attention deficit problems, to name but
a few.*

*All problems have emotional and psychological aspects.
These can be readily addressed using TFT. Other
significant benefits are that there are no side effects,
which, alas, cannot be said of much of conventional
medicine. Another important factor is that no belief
or faith is required on the part of the patient. These
techniques work. When patients notice significant
improvement or resolution of their problems, they are
often surprised and mystified, and try to find alternative
explanations as to why they are better, not believing
that a sequence of taps can have had such a significant
effect on problems which have often been present for a
long time.*

TFT also addresses the issue of Psychological Reversal. This is not addressed by conventional medicine, but is often the stumbling block which has caused other approaches to fail. This is identified and treated thoroughly and efficiently by TFT, enabling progress to be made where previously there had been only frustration.

Patients often have an awareness of the effect of dietary constituents and environmental factors on their health. These people are significantly vulnerable, as conventional medicine has little to offer, once genuine allergic disease has been excluded. However, these environmental toxins can be identified and their effects treated with great accuracy using TFT.

TFT is a great addition to a doctor's toolkit. It is safe, easy to learn and, more importantly, simple to practise. I have found that the more I employ TFT techniques with patients, the more areas emerge where it may be even more helpful. What a doctor requires to employ TFT is an open mind: to be prepared to be surprised. While dealing with the presenting problem is often simple and swift, very frequently patients notice all sorts of other issues in their life take on a different light after TFT treatment, and new ways forward emerge in all sorts of areas, apparently unrelated to the problem they sought advice for in the first place. I find the analogy to peeling an onion highly appropriate. The presenting problem is the outer layer. Once that is addressed and peeled away, the next layer emerges. This may be what was being sought, in which case the job is done, or it may require some intervention in its own right. As progress is made, the nearer the patient comes to finding the healthy centre.

To quote Stephen Tovey, author of The Seven Habits of Highly Successful People, *it is very important to 'start with the end in mind'. Once an objective or series of objectives has been negotiated and agreed with the patient, what is required then are very sensitive and accurate calibration skills. Thus a constant check can be kept that progress is being made in the appropriate direction, or the necessary adjustments identified and made. These negotiating and calibration skills are an essential part of the skill set necessary for general practice, and when used with TFT, excellent results rapidly follow.*

I have some very simple rules of engagement when people approach me requesting TFT. These are an extension of my rules for any successful intervention, conventional or otherwise.

The first is that the patient is not seeking TFT as an alternative to conventional medicine for a problem which could significantly deteriorate if appropriate conventional treatment is unnecessarily delayed. As a GP I am in a good position to help them decide this.

Secondly, the patient must be coming to me for help of his or her own free will. If patients are coming because they are being sent by someone else, for whatever reason, the outcome is likely to be disappointing at best.

Thirdly, the patient takes responsibility for the outcome. As part of the TFT intervention, I will give the patient some drills to follow regularly. These reinforce and strengthen the progress made, and are crucial to achieving the desired result.

The final word goes to Dr Roger Callahan, the genius who developed Thought Field Therapy and who, even though now well into his ninth decade, continues to develop new applications for the technology he discovered. In his teaching Dr Callahan says that any therapist who claims 100 per cent success for any intervention has not treated enough people. TFT is swift and effective. It achieves results often where other approaches have failed to do so. Typically only one or two appointments are necessary for any particular issue. TFT also complements eloquently and adds to the successes achieved by other forms of intervention. It can do no harm, and can often produce quick results when none looked possible.

Dr Mark Chambers

How Toxic Are You?

A few times throughout this book, I have mentioned the term 'toxins'. What I mean by these are Individual Energy Toxins or IETs. These are quite different to the word 'toxin' in its traditional sense, which typically relates to substances that are harmful to everyone, such as arsenic, lead or mercury. An IET may be ostensibly a healthy substance such as cranberry juice, but for certain individuals may be 'toxic' in its effect. Not only can IETs block TFT treatment, but they can have a devastating effect on your overall wellbeing.

The chances are you are not functioning at an optimal level, perhaps emotionally or physically, or both, even though you may not even know it. If you have only ever functioned at 50 per cent of your potential, then that is what you perceive as 'as good as it gets' because you don't know any better. This chapter may improve your 'vitality' beyond recognition.

You may be reacting to things that you eat, potions or lotions that you put on your body, or substances that you inhale such as perfume or air fresheners, which are like energy vampires: they literally drain you of emotional and physical energy. That is the power of an IET. Because you may not know what they are, they are insidious and silent in the ways they act, until one day you notice you don't have the energy some other people have, or that you used to have.

Symptoms of recurring use of IETs – in no particular order:

- **malaise**
- **sticky faeces**

- ongoing anxiety
- insomnia
- irritability
- lack of focus/concentration
- poor memory
- cravings
- red or itchy skin
- fatigue after meals
- bowel irregularity, constipation or diarrhoea
- unexplained or magnified aches and pains
- increased congestion
- amplified emotions/tearfulness
- stress
- regular unexplained headaches.

And the list goes on …

You may already be familiar with the term 'allergen', which is the name given to any substance that you have an allergic reaction to. Allergic reactions have two forms:

1. **IgE response – this is immediate and, often, extreme. After consumption of the offending substance the individual experiences a debilitating physical reaction as the body releases histamine and other chemicals at a rapid rate, often within seconds or possibly up to 2 hours later; this can cause symptoms such as a chronic rash, coughing and wheezing, or anaphylaxis, where the mouth and throat swell and death can result from the inability to breathe. Thankfully, these reactions are very rare.**
2. **IgG response – this is a delayed reaction caused by the overproduction of antibodies to a specific allergen, which**

Welcome to Rushden Library
rushlib@northamptonshire.gov.uk
www.northamptonshire.gov.uk/renew

Title: Great tales from English history :Cheddar
Man to
ID: 00400820730

Title: Tapping for life :how to eliminate negative
thou
ID: 80003140556

Title: David and Goliath :underdogs, misfits and
the ar
ID: 80003341718

Title: What do we really know? :the big
questions of ph
ID: 80003281894

Title: Great tales from English history
ID: 00400910781

Title: Dr right all along
ID: 00401042759

Title: Cattle baron needs a bride
ID: 00400995938

Title: Pregnant - father wanted
ID: 00400985468

Total items: 8
02/08/2014 13:17

bind to the allergen and enter the bloodstream. This challenges the immune system and can cause a number of symptoms, similar in nature to the response to an IET. Often when a migraine sufferer consumes an IET they will experience migraine symptoms anything up to 48 hours later.

Both of these responses can be measured with a simple blood test. The difference between these and an IET is that you cannot measure a response to a perfume, for example, with a blood test. Ingested IETs may also not show up in a blood test as they affect the body on an 'energy' level rather than a measurable physiological level.

The good news is that, for most people, IETs can be measured using the same applied kinesiology test described on page 53. This is because we are testing to see what substances affect our energy, and this is clearly demonstrated using the muscle test.

If you suffer from ongoing anxiety, OCD or any other chronic emotional problem, then it is likely you are consuming, either by ingesting or inhaling, one or more IETs on a regular basis. Identifying and removing them from your diet/lifestyle can be totally liberating and life-changing.

The Toxin Barrel

Just like the concept of an emotional barrel we talked about earlier, in the same way you also have a toxin barrel. Of course we are all exposed to IETs every day: when we walk down the street we inhale car fumes which are IETs for everyone, i.e. known toxins, and we have a filtration system that enables us to cope with a small level of toxicity. The problem occurs when you unknowingly consume IETs, perhaps daily. The effects can be devastating.

How to Test for Toxins

Unfortunately, when looking at ingested toxins it is often the things we like or crave most of all that cause a problem. If you have an ongoing emotional issue such as anxiety or OCD, then keep a food diary for a week and also note when you feel lowest in terms of energy, and suffer from the most anxiety. Then look at the foods you eat and see if there's a pattern.

The first thing to do is to identify whether there is one particular food you eat. For example, if you have wholewheat cereal for breakfast, a roll for lunch and pasta for tea, then wheat features too heavily in your diet! With my 'nutritionist' head on, I believe there's often a point at which your body says 'enough!' of a specific food, and you may become intolerant to it simply because you consume too much of it and have done for some time. This may or may not be the case with IETs, but what you eat most of is the best place to start testing. The good news is that if you find something you eat a lot of *is* an IET, and you remove it from your diet, by virtue of the fact that you consumed it every day and you felt bad every day, eliminating it can totally transform your energy levels.

Here's a reminder of how the arm test works and the words to use. In this example I will use 'wheat', but of course you name whatever the food is you are testing:

1. **Calibrate and check for Psychological Reversal (PR). When you have a strong arm with palm down and a weak arm**

with palm up, you can proceed. If you detect a reversal, then BOTH you and the person helping you must correct for PR (see page 60).

2. Identify the food to be tested and hold the 'thought' of it clearly in your mind. Even better: if you have it to hand, hold it and place your hand on the centre of your chest.

3. Say 'wheat' while your partner arm-tests you:
   • If the arm stays strong, move to the next stage (4); if the arm goes weak, you are toxic for wheat and should remove it from your diet.

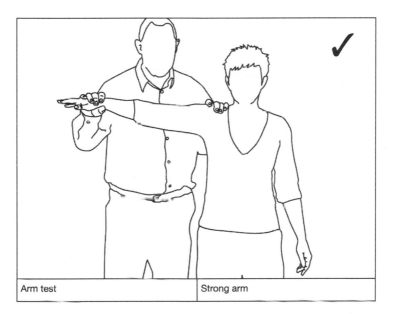

| Arm test | Strong arm |

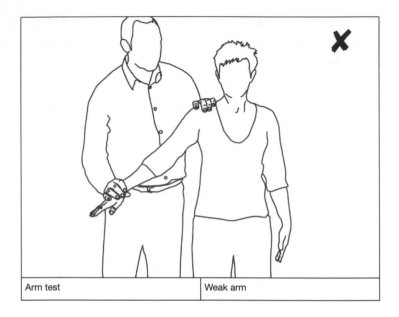

Arm test	Weak arm

4. Say 'wheat, I want to be healthy' while your partner arm-tests you:
   - If the arm stays strong, move to the next stage (5); if the arm goes weak, you are toxic for wheat and should remove it from your diet.
5. Say 'wheat, I want to be sick':
   - If the arm is weak, and the two previous statements were strong, then the wheat is NOT toxic for you.
   - If the arm is strong you are in psychological reversal; clear this using the corrective treatments as follows:
   - Tap side hand (**sh**) – check for sore spot (**ss**) and rub gently if located – tap under nose (**un**).
6. Repeat the test from the beginning. It is likely the food will prove toxic to you.

Note: If you get a weak arm when it should be strong, it may be the tester who is reversed, so at all times BOTH of you must do the PR corrections.

What to Do If the Item Is Toxic

The food needs to bo removed from your diet completely and totally, ideally permanently. In the event that what you are diagnosing is a substance that initiates an IgG response, you MAY be able to reintroduce it in small amounts after 3–4 months, but you should never go back to consuming it in the same amounts. It will be a case of little and not very often. In any event, STOP having the food completely and in any form for 3–4 months, then retest.

What If You Can't Get a Clear Arm Test or Don't Have Anyone to Help You?

Although it works for almost everyone, occasionally some people are very difficult to arm-test and in this instance results can be unreliable or difficult to interpret. In this case, TFT Voice Technology is the best option for you.

You should only use a *registered* Voice Technology therapist (see the details in the Further Resources chapter). Your voice can then be analysed and, as you name foods or other substances, your VT therapist will be able to measure your resistance or otherwise to the item and give you immediate and accurate results.

Toxins and TFT Treatments

As I have mentioned several times, if carried out in the correct manner exactly as I have described in this book, TFT has a success rate of between 70 and 80 per cent. If you are part of the minority of people it does not work for, you may need to seek the help of a TFT diagnostic therapist (TFT-Dx) or, for more complicated cases, a Voice Technology (VT) therapist.

If a treatment is not working, there are a few things you can try first:

- **Check you are in the thought field.**
- **Check you are using the correct algorithm or sequence and following the correct protocol.**
- **Check for and clear reversals using corrective treatments including cb2 if needed.**
- **Check for toxins.**

Once you have identified a toxin, it needs to be cleared from your system. Typically the method for doing that is advanced TFT and beyond the scope of this book, however there is a treatment that may help in the first instance:

1. **Tap the index finger 20+ times, tap side hand 20+ times.**
2. **Do cb2 while thinking about the substance.**

Repeat the initial treatment protocol.

If these two steps do not work there is no point continuing as it will only lead to frustration. You need to eliminate the toxin for at least a week, doing cb2 at least twice per day and tapping **sh** regularly, and then do the treatment again. If you have had seven days staying out of PR and your body is beginning to clear the IET naturally, there is a chance it will allow treatment to be successful.

>>>Joanne's Story

Some time ago I had a call from a lovely woman in Cornwall who needed treating for 24/7 anxiety. She could not get to either my London or Leicester clinic easily, so I did some work with her over the phone and ultimately referred her to Sean Quigley for VT. She had two sessions in which Sean cleared a number of past issues and traumas and identified quite a few toxins, typically wheat.

I spoke to Joanne after the treatment and she was most disappointed that she had not experienced the miraculous results she had predicted from the TFT, having been recommended it by a friend who had had exactly that result. She was very reluctant to stop eating wheat and could not understand how that could possibly affect her emotionally. Actually, she was quite cross!

Six months later I received a lovely email saying how she had woken up one day and realized that for the past few days she had no felt anxiety at all. It had completely gone. She had, it seems, decided that giving up on wheat was worth a try, and cut it out. Within two weeks her energy levels started to improve and after three months all her anxiety had gone. She then cautiously began to have a little wheat occasionally, and the anxiety had stayed away. Her life was transformed. The miraculous cure she had hoped for became a reality; it just took a little longer than expected!

As mentioned earlier, Voice Technology (VT) TFT is a highly specialized treatment. Algorithm-level practitioners often refer on complicated cases to a VT practitioner, and Sean

Quigley is one such highly respected and highly skilled VT practitioner who works daily with clients like this. Often the reason the standard TFT treatment does not work is due to IETs, and here I have asked Sean to share his thoughts on IETs with you:

> 'The discovery that energy toxins influence our emotions, health and general wellbeing has required me to review drastically not only the way I treat my clients and the order of things, but the view I take on everything in, on and around our bodies, including my own.
>
> 'Many of my clients have seen dramatic changes in the way they feel as they have come to understand the negative effects for them personally caused directly by IETs; and by removing them from their diet or their environment, they have been able to restore their emotional and physical health.
>
> 'My findings are that IETs affect so many areas of our lives; as a VT practitioner I am often working with the 10–15 per cent of clients for whom traditional TFT and all other forms of treatment have not worked, and this is almost always due to them having a very large and full or even overflowing 'toxin barrel'. It is common that once I have diagnosed and cleared IETs, a TFT treatment can be carried out effectively and with immediate benefits.
>
> 'As part of my VT work I treat many clients with chronic emotional and/or physical problems, such as ME, MS, depression, ADHD, even cancer and other life-threatening diseases. By diagnosing and eliminating

toxins, clients can stay out of PR (Psychological Reversal) and allow the body to perform its inbuilt natural healing function. Toxins can hold us in a negative PR state, which not only amplifies our emotional problems, turning a normal slight concern into a full-blown panic attack, for example, but it can severely hamper our natural physical healing process as well. The benefits of identifying and removing IETs include new levels of energy, the removal of tired spells and the need for afternoon catnaps; this brings freedom from excessive emotional outbursts or abnormally amplified anxiety, irrational outbursts and various levels of depression including ADHD and ADD. Arthritis and other pains can simply go away once the IETs are identified and removed.

'In my own life, I had always suffered unexplained periods of doziness, especially after meals, which I always put down to erratic blood-sugar levels. Once I cleared my toxins, however, my energy levels increased dramatically, I no longer had bloating and stomach pains, and my dyslexia, which has been a challenge all my life, all but disappeared. It was a stunning transformation; I now wake up with a high level of energy that is sustained throughout the day.
VT is NOT a cure, but as a diagnostic method and treatment tool it is invaluable, as it allows clients to understand and achieve their optimum state, both physically and emotionally. It is crucial that we seriously consider IE toxins and their associated debilitating effects when we judge the effectiveness of TFT, and, if diagnosed, adjust our lifestyles accordingly'.

– Sean Quigley, TFT-VT

Algorithm Table: The Sequences You Need to Help Yourself to Health

The following table shows the algorithms as created by Dr Callahan and as taught at basic Algorithm-level training sessions. You will notice, specifically in the later chapters which deal with treating specific problems, that there are some additional sequences that I have developed based on understanding the emotion attached to the meridian point and correctly diagnosing the sequence, either after detailed conversations with a client and eliciting the emotions involved in 'the problem', or by using traditional diagnostic (Dx) methods which form part of Advanced TFT Training. For clarity and to avoid confusion, these additional *algos* are NOT included in this table.

How to Use this Table

The first column lists the 'problem' or emotion/s; the second column is the number of the *algo*. This makes it easier to refer to if you remember the individual number of the *algo* rather than the whole sequence. The third column lists the tapping sequence (the *algo* itself).

As shown in the protocol, ALL *algos* involve first tapping the sequence (majors), then the **9g,** then repeating the sequence. This is written as **e a c 9g sq**, with **9g** meaning 9 gamut and **sq** meaning 'repeat the sequence' (the majors). When the SUD is 2 or less, then always finish with the eye roll (**er**).

SUD readings are taken continually. Refer back to pages 38–39 often until you are totally confident with the process.

You will notice that some *algos* are much longer than others, depending on the complexity of the problem. Some are as short as one point.

Notice also that in some cases there is more than one *algo*, for example, for an addictive urge (5–8) and panic/anxiety disorder (29–34) you may need to try the different variations until you find the one that works best for you.

You will also notice that some *algos* are the same, for example, 1 and 4. The reason that the same *algo* can work for treating different emotional states is that you are in a different thought field.

Most *algos* are for emotional issues, but there are *algos* for physical pain and also for jetlag and clumsiness (which is usually a symptom of reversal).

Remember that for any given problem you may need to use several *algos* as you peel away the layers. It's unlikely with a complex past trauma, for example, that one *algo* will clear all aspects of the problem. You may clear the trauma aspect of the event with one *algo*, and need another one for anger, and another for sadness, etc. As long as you work in stages, are systematic in your approach and keep it simple, then you are likely to be successful in most cases.

If you do choose the wrong *algo*, YOU WILL DO NO HARM; it just will not work. This gives you the freedom to try different *algos* safely until you find the one that works best for you.

Most simple phobias/fear	1	e a c 9g sq
Spider phobia/claustrophobia/fear of turbulence in flight	2	a e c 9g sq
	3	e c a c e 9g sq
General anxiety/stress	4	e a c 9g sq
Addictive urge	5	c e c
	6	e a c 9g sq
	7	a e c 9g sq
	8	e c a c 9g sq
Simple trauma/rejection/love pain/grief	9	eb c 9g sq
Complex trauma/rejection/love pain/grief	10	eb e a c 9g sq
Complex trauma with guilt	11	eb e a c if c 9g sq
Complex trauma with anger	12	eb e a c tf 9g sq
Intimidation	13	eb e un c if 9g sq
Jealousy	14	mf a c 9g sq
Guilt	15	if c 9g sq
Anger	16	tf c 9g sq
Frustration/impatience	17	eb e a c tf c 9g sq
Rage	18	oe c 9g sq
Obsession/OCD	19	c e c 9q sq
	20	e a c 9g sq
	21	a e c 9g sq
	22	e c a c 9g sq
Depression	23	g50 c 9g sq
Complex depression	24	eb oe e un ul a c tf if 9g sq
Physical pain	25	g50 c 9g sq
	26	eb e g50 9g sq
Embarrassment	27	un 9g sq
Shame	28	ul 9g sq
Panic/anxiety disorder	29	eb e a c 9g sq
	30	e a eb c tf 9g sq

	31	a e eb c tf 9g sq
	32	eb a e 9g sq
	33	e eb a tf 9g sq
	34	c e a 9g sq
Jet lag (East–West)	35	a c 9g sq
Jet lag (West–East)	36	e c 9g sq
For the inability to visualize, overcome addictions or achieve peak performance	37	a c 9g sq
Enhancement of motivation	38	e c e 9g sq
Self-sabotage/negative behaviour	39	Correct for various levels of PR as shown previously (page 60)
Reversal of concepts, words or behaviours	40	Correct for various levels of PR as shown previously (page 60)
Abnormal clumsiness or awkwardness	41	Collarbone breathing (cb2)
When SUD is 2 or less		Eye roll

Spend some time looking at the *algos* and referring back to the table showing which meridian tapping point relates to which specific emotion, and you will begin to understand the reason for certain sequences. Of course this is not necessary for it to work! You can just hold the thought and follow the tapping protocol, blissfully ignorant of any of the meanings of the sequences, and it will still work. If you are sceptical and don't think it will work, it makes NO difference to the success rate. Providing you are in the thought, not reversed and using the relevant sequence, is it likely to work even for the most sceptical non-believer; although he or she is most likely to suffer from the Apex problem!

This brings to an end the general information and technical guidelines for TFT; if you have read through so far thoroughly and followed the exercises, you will by now be able to use TFT to good general effect to eliminate most negative emotions in most cases.

The good news is that there's even more helpful stuff to come; the next chapter looks at how Neuro-Linguistic Programming (NLP) can be used to replace those negative emotions with good feelings and instal new behaviours and 'programming' that will enable you to be free from your problems and create new resourceful states and patterns.

TFT and NLP are the perfect couple.

As you know now, TFT is awesome at eliminating most negative thoughts and feelings for most people. Having removed 'the problem' it can leave quite a void, especially if someone has had the problem for some time and got used to behaving and thinking in a certain (negative) way. The brain likes what it knows, and sometimes we do what we know because it's familiar and that makes it comfortable even if it isn't that good or that enjoyable for us – and sometimes even if it's bad! Fear of the unknown is a pretty strong emotion; there's a security in consistency. When you have removed a problem or a negative behaviour that you have had for some time with TFT, then the icing on the cake is to use NLP to replace the old, negative feelings with some new, positive ones. This is where NLP comes into its own.

Part 3
Replacing Negative Thoughts with New, Positive Ones

How Your Brain Works

Before we explore NLP, and how it can help you to change your mind, let's take a basic look at how your brain works.

The brain is a truly amazing structure which, as a result of its process, defines who you are and how you experience the world. It is made up of several components and its appearance to the naked eye is that of wobbly, wrinkly tubes all moulded together to make a shape that fits within the skill. It is a somewhat mystical organ, in that we cannot see within its anatomical structure and observe its workings in the same way as we can, for example, with the lungs. When I was taught biology at school I was told to imagine the inside of the lungs as an upside-down tree. The oxygen comes in through the 'trunk' and is then diverted into large 'branches' then smaller 'twigs' and finally into the leaves (which represent the alveoli in the lungs) and are very fine (only one cell thick), and it is here that the oxygen passes through and the carbon dioxide is picked up. The carbon dioxide then makes the journey in reverse, through the twigs into the branches, up the trunk and out through the mouth. It makes perfect sense, and all these structures can be observed and the alveoli dissected.

When you look inside the brain, however, there is a more complex structure; and because you can't 'see' thoughts or feelings, you cannot trace them in the way that you can trace the flow of oxygen or carbon dioxide within the lungs. Mechanically, specialists can locate which part of the brain moves certain limbs, for example, but when it comes to thoughts, emotions or feelings it's less clear; yet your highly unique view of the world lies not in the mechanical workings of your brain, but in some invisible chemistry we have only just begun to understand.

One of the key aspects of the brain is that it operates both 'consciously' and 'unconsciously'. On a conscious level we can process (plus or minus two) seven pieces of information at any time. As you read this now, think about the words you are reading and how you are learning, maybe you are aware of an internal voice in your head reading out the words to you, maybe you are aware of how the pages of the book feel beneath your hands, how you are sitting or lying. Now place your attention on the largest toe on your right foot, notice how you can think about that now, and be fully aware of how it feels, yet were previously completely unaware of it on a conscious level; yet if while you were reading someone came along with a lit match and held it under your toe, your brain would instantaneously receive the message that it needed to move the toe immediately. Prior to the match your brain was quietly monitoring your toe and how it felt in your unconscious mind. You were unaware of this, yet if there were a significant and potentially dangerous change, an urgent message would be sent. This is the case for all of your body, not just externally but your inner physiological workings as well. They are under unconscious control. Via a complex system of feedback your heart knows how often to beat, your lungs know at which rate to breathe, your kidneys know how to adapt to achieve correct blood pressure and blood pH, and numerous other functions are all kept under control.

In practical terms, when you walk into a supermarket and go down the aisles, your unconscious processes every single product on every shelf, every person you pass along the way, all the sounds, changes in temperature and smells in different aisles. You process more information unconsciously than you can possibly imagine in your conscious mind.

If you have ever seen the movie *Bruce Almighty* with Jim Carrey and Morgan Freeman, remember the scene when Bruce is with God, and God is telling Bruce how it feels to hear all the prayers of all the people from all over the world coming in at any one time. God then turns up the volume of what he hears and puts it on speaker so Bruce can hear it as well. The result is an immense number of sounds coming through from millions of different voices in a range of languages, all with their own message. Bruce of course falls to the ground clutching his ears as he cannot comprehend processing that level of information. The sound of all these prayers represents all the signals, internally and externally, that your unconscious is processing every second. Wow!

If you think of your mind as a huge iceberg, with only the top peeping out above the waterline, then your conscious mind would be that small peak, and the body of it under the water is your unconscious. Depending which research you read, your unconscious represents approximately 90–95 per cent of your thinking and processing.

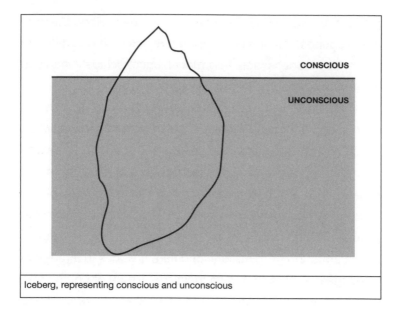

Iceberg, representing conscious and unconscious

When it comes to learning, you learn by consciously receiving and processing information through your five senses:

1. **Smell**
2. **Touch**
3. **Taste**
4. **Sight**
5. **Sound.**

Your brain then assimilates this information and reaches a conclusion, based largely on associations, which then determine your subsequent actions. If you continue to process information in the same way and reach the same conclusions, then you create a 'pattern' or a learned behaviour. Once this pattern is accepted into your unconscious mind, then it becomes effectively 'installed', and whenever you are in this situation this response becomes your 'default setting'. A simple example of this might be if as a child whenever you cried or were upset your mum said, 'Stop crying and you can have a biscuit.' You'd then associate having a biscuit with being comforted. This pattern is repeated often enough that it becomes a default behaviour and you 'automatically' reach for a biscuit whenever you are upset. You can develop and expand this behaviour further by including any similar confectionery! It may be reinforced by images of *Bridget Jones* or *Friends* characters shown tucking into a tub of ice cream or a bar of chocolate when their characters are fed up or depressed, looking for comfort; the advertising agencies are well aware of these learned behaviours and play to them in their marketing campaigns.

The good news is that you can 'unlearn' these patterns by literally changing your mind.

The brain is divided into two hemispheres, right and left. Each has its own characteristics and processes information in different ways. Most people have a dominant side; however, to achieve optimum levels of brain functioning, learning to use both hemispheres equally and in balance is essential. When you can achieve this, learning is enhanced and you have more resources in terms of how you process information and the choices you make.

A left-brain-dominant person is likely to process information in a linear fashion, i.e. from start to finish in logical steps, 'chunking down' information and piecing it together in the correct order. Very systematic, a left-brainer uses the information received and processes it in a precise order.

Left-brainers are great list-makers; they are also usually good spellers, as this involves sequencing; they also give directions in a very specific order of sequence and detail. They also typically articulate very well how they feel, finding the precise words necessary to convey their feelings. When left-brainers are faced with a change in environment, they adapt to it logically. They like order; a good example of an extreme left-brainer is Monica in *Friends*.

A right-brainer, in contrast, likes to know the outcome in advance and see the 'bigger picture' before they start. They work best when they understand what's at stake conceptually and can then create a system to achieve a given goal, which is not necessarily logical in its format. Right-brainers are more random in their processing and may flit from one task to another, getting the same amount done as a left-brainer but in a completely different way. The right side of the brain is colour-sensitive and very kinaesthetic, it likes to see, feel or touch; right-brainers often know what they want to say but cannot find the exact words to convey it, as a feeling is not tangible. Right-brainers are creative and artistic compared to left-brainers, who are more digital (that is, analytical in the way they process information). You are more likely to find a right-brainer involved in television production or the entertainment industry, and more likely to find a left-brainer as an accountant or engineer. An example of a right-brainer is Phoebe in *Friends*.

All of this information can be used to good advantage when you want to change your mind, as we will see with some of the exercises I will show you later on.

The Discovery of NLP

Richard Bandler and John Grinder are described as the creators of NLP, but in reality what they achieved was more of a discovery. Imagine an intrepid explorer searching for treasure: he or she studies maps, learns about the geology of the area and the history of events, and pays attention to the most minute detail, processing all of this knowledge along with a vivacious curiosity and love of the subject. As a result he or she is 'lucky' enough to find the treasure.

We all have our own treasure or 'lost city of Atlantis' within us. Because we may not have found it yet, this does not mean it does not exist. We need to be intrepid explorers of our own destiny, and NLP can be our guide. To my mind, Bandler and Grinder are intrepid explorers who shared their discoveries with all who showed a genuine interest. During their searches they documented and analysed all they found, and used that knowledge to replicate it. For them, the 'city of Atlantis' that they explored comprised a collection of highly skilled and successful therapists, all of whom were unique and somewhat non-conformist in their methods. They assessed these methodologies in the smallest detail and modelled them.

If you want to make an exceedingly good cake, a really excellent exceedingly good cake, you have several options which would have varying degrees of success:

- **get the ingredients and have a go at guessing the correct amounts and techniques**
- **get a recipe book, select a recipe and follow the instructions**

- if your very favourite cake is, for example, a Kipling cake, then go and spend a day with Mr Kipling and watch him make a cake, really observing in the most minute detail so that you can repeat exactly the same process yourself afterwards.

It's pretty clear which is likely to have the best outcome in terms of how you develop your skills.

Bandler and Grinder, through observation and the study of their work, modelled successful therapists of their time, most prominently Milton Erikson, Virginia Satir and Fritz Perls, in order to understand and replicate their methods and use that information as a basis from which to develop and adapt these techniques further.

Milton Erikson

Milton Erikson was a world-renowned hypnotherapist who was physically crippled by polio, and who developed an amazing capacity for observing other people's behaviour, particularly as represented in their language and what they said about how they felt. By using and reflecting back certain language patterns, he was able to get subjects to think and process in a different way, both in hypnotically-induced trance and in what became known as 'conversational hypnosis'. Eriksonian hypnosis is now taught as a method of hypnosis in its own right, and Eriksonian language often deliberately juxtaposes certain words in order to cause the brain to experience confusion and subsequently question its thinking processes. This has proven to be a highly effective method of change-work.

Virginia Satir

Virginia Satir was a psychotherapist who specialized in working with families. At the time her belief that 'the presenting idea is seldom the real problem' was considered a novel approach. Her work, in particular in the area of self-esteem and family communication and interaction, defined her and set her apart as an elite therapist. She wrote many books and received the American Association for Marriage and Family Therapy's Distinguished Service Award in 1973. She used humour and made physical visual representations by asking people to stand or sit in a certain way to demonstrate their feelings externally. Using these and other tools, such as role-play, she was able to create a safe place so that people could open themselves up to new experiences. This was a new way of working and one which has now been adopted into many 'modern' psychological methods.

The quotation at the start of this book was taken from a book by Virginia Satir called *Meditations and Inspirations*; and you will find another excerpt in later chapters.

Fritz Perls

Fritz Perls was a German psychoanalyst who fled with his wife Laura to South Africa to escape Nazi oppression and subsequently moved to New York after the Second World War. They worked together and used role-play and other active techniques in a therapeutic role, which later became known as Gestalt therapy. The emphasis of Gestalt therapy is not on the client's past experiences, although these are acknowledged, but focuses more intently on how it affects the client NOW. In this way clients are guided through 'unfinished business' and taught to accept their individual complexities fully, to free themselves from past pain and anxiety and low self-esteem, and develop in a way appropriate for them.

Bandler identified language patterns used by Perls which he believed enhanced the effectiveness of Gestalt therapy.

Modalities

Of course Bandler and Grinder not only modelled the therapists; they also looked carefully at the clients' responses to treatments and noticed many commonalities in the way we assimilate, process and encode information, both verbally and, more importantly, with non-verbal responses. One of the early 'discoveries' they made was that we have essentially three modalities, or filters, through which we process information. We all use all three, but there is a tendency to be dominant in one. This can be very restrictive in terms of our options and choices, and in the same way that balancing right and left brain can optimize our performance, opening up our *visual, auditory* and *kinaesthetic* 'portals' can greatly enhance our functioning on many levels. In NLP these are called our *representation systems* or *submodalities*. This list of modalities can also be further increased to include olfactory (smell) and gustatory (taste) filters.

In this book I will concentrate on techniques that enable you to communicate better with yourself. Your internal dialogue or 'inner voice' is probably the most influential part of your day-to-day processing. We often speak to ourselves in a scathing or insulting way, which we would never use with our friends or anyone at all we care about. And we let ourselves get away with it!

Be careful what you say – you might be listening.

There are certain words that indicate a specific submodality/
representation system:

VISUAL	AUDITORY	KINAESTHETIC	OLFACTORY	GUSTATORY
See	Hear	Feel	Smell	Taste
Look	Listen	Touch	Aroma	Bitter
Focus	Tune in	Grasp	Bouquet	Bland
Show	Sound wave	Hold	Stench	Sharp
Appear	Wavelength	Pressure	Rotten	Sweet
Picture	Talk	Push	Putrid	Sour
Bright	Say	Hard	Musty	Spicy
Image	Discuss	Hot		Tangy
Clear	Noisy	Cold		
Perspective	Silence	Cool		
Hazy	Resonate	Rub		
Sparkling	Shout	Firm		
Flash	Quiet	Tense		
Glimpse	Click	Concrete		
Colourful	Speak	Solid		
Vague	Chatter	Flow		
Horizon	Volume	Heavy		
Hindsight	Utter	Hunch		
Clarity	Sound	Shift		
Watch	Earshot	Tension		
– and many more	Mention	– and many more		
...	– and many more	...		
	...			

The following assessment is based on one used by Rod
Piggott from the College of Transformational Therapy. Rod
trained me in clinical hypnosis. The ranges looked at in this test
are: visual, auditory, kinaesthetic and digital (left-brained).

For each of the following statements, place a number
next to it using the following guidelines:

4 = closest to describing you

3 = next best description

2 = next best

1 = least describes you

	QUESTION 1	SCORE
	I make important decisions based on:	
1	Gut-level feelings and instinct	
2	What sounds best	
3	What I see is the best	
4	Precise review and analysis of all options	

	QUESTION 2	SCORE
	During an argument I am likely to be influenced by:	
1	The other person's tone of voice	
2	Whether or not I can see their point of view	
3	The logic of their argument	
4	Whether or not I feel they are honest and understand their feelings	

	QUESTION 3	SCORE
	I most easily communicate what is going on with me by:	
1	The way I dress and look	
2	The feelings I share	
3	The words I choose	
4	The tone of my voice	

	QUESTION 4	SCORE
	It is easiest for me to:	
1	Find the ideal volume on a stereo	
2	Select the most intellectually relevant point on a given subject	
3	Select the most comfortable furniture, e.g. bed, sofa or armchair	
4	Select rich, attractive colourful combinations	

	QUESTION 5	SCORE
	I am very:	
1	Attuned to the sounds in my surroundings	
2	Adept at making sense of facts and data	
3	Sensitive to how clothes feel on my skin	
4	Responsive to the colours and design in a room	

Scoring

Step 1: Copy your answers from the test to the boxes below in the exact same sequence: for example, if for Q1 the order of your answers was 4-3-2-1, complete as follows:

Example:

Q1
K 4
A 3
V 2
D 1

Q1	Q2	Q3	Q4	Q5
K	A	V	A	A
A	V	K	D	D
V	D	D	K	K
D	K	A	V	V

Step 2: Using the box below, fill in the numbers/scores associated with each letter. There will be five entries for each letter – for example, if for Q1 you gave V a 2, write 2 in the first box.

Example of Q1 (where your answers were 4-3-2-1).

QUESTION	V	K	A	D
1	2	4	3	1
2				
3				
4				
5				
TOTAL				

Total up your scores. The totals will indicate your preference for each representational system. If you have a huge difference between your top score and the others, then you will benefit enormously as you begin to consider using your other filters, at first intentionally and then, after a while, automatically.

Changing Behaviour

When you want to change a behaviour or learn a new skill, you first have to acknowledge the old behaviour which you are so used to that you don't even realize it no longer serves you any purpose. Let's say, for example, that when you are 'doing' depression you make images in your mind that are very dark. You physically keep your head down and drop your shoulders, your internal voice is very negative, pointing out the worst that could happen, etc. I doubt very much that (unless you have studied NLP) you have ever thought consciously about how you 'do' depression.

There is a great model for explaining how things become 'habits' – in other words, the process you go through before something becomes your 'default setting'. If you have passed your driving test and have been driving for some time, think about the first lesson you ever had: trying to feel for the 'bite' of the clutch, listening to the change in revs in the engine so you know when to change gear, remembering to look in the rear-view mirror, sensing the feel of the accelerator and the brake underneath your feet, having to move your feet simultaneously when you brake so that you don't stall, the mirror-signal-manoeuvre sequence – you were processing so much information consciously as you learned these techniques. After a few lessons you began to sense automatically what to do and when, but you were still thinking consciously about what to do – especially on your test! Think about how you drive now; have you ever been driving and thought 'Where am I?' or 'How did I get here?' Especially if it's a journey you have done many times. When I ran health clubs I had a 40-minute drive home from work, and after a long day I often got to a point where I didn't know which village I had just passed through. I had been driving safely, but on an unconscious level. You might call it automatic pilot.

Have you ever been around someone who genuinely believes they are good at something they are dreadful at? They are completely oblivious to it. You only have to watch the early rounds of the *X Factor* to see this in evidence – people who genuinely believe they can do something well that they are actually very bad at. This is called *unconscious incompetence*.

Then you have people who are bad at something and acknowledge they are bad at it. They know they cannot do it, they don't need to be told. This is called *conscious incompetence*. When you have this level of acceptance, you can begin to change.

When you start to learn a new skill or a new behaviour, but have to think about it as you do it, as with driving, then you become *consciously competent*. This simply means you can do it when you think about it.

After a while and some considerable repetition, this behaviour becomes *automatic*; you can do it without thinking. You can drive from A to B chatting away or listening to the radio, singing along, changing gear and doing all your checks instinctively. This is when you become *unconsciously competent.*

When Bandler and Grinder modelled Erikson, Satir and Perls, they were watching people who were exceptional in their field, who were unconsciously competent. Interestingly, they themselves didn't even know why they were so good at what they did. When Erikson was presented with the 'breakdown' of his communication and techniques, he allegedly said, 'So *that's* how I do it' ... or so the story goes.

There is another level above unconsciously competent: *unconscious mastery*. This is where you perform something really well without any thought or effort. There's a famous story of when Laurence Olivier, after giving a truly outstanding performance of *Hamlet*, after a 20-minute standing ovation went into his dressing room very frustrated. His dresser asked him how he could be anything other than delighted as he had just given *the* best performance of Hamlet ever. Olivier said he knew that, and the reason he was so cross was that he had absolutely no idea how he had done it!

Many sports professionals also achieve this level of mastery. Tiger Woods, for example, is a great example of 'getting into the zone' of unconscious mastery. Some people who experience this level of mastery describe it as an almost spiritual experience.

Why is this important? Actually, it's *essential*, because if you 'do' depression, then you need to learn how to 'do' happy instead. If you are so good at doing depression – that is, if you are unconsciously competent at doing depression, then the first step is in acknowledging that it is a thought process, and that if you use different thought processes you will get a different outcome.

While TFT can beautifully remove the cause of the depression, it's a good idea to learn how to programme your mind to STOP doing depression. I am going to teach you some basic techniques that will enable you to do this.

Before we go any further, I want you to read through the following exercise, then stand up and do it before you carry on reading. It's just a few easy steps:

1. **Stand up and lift your dominant arm out in front of you and point forwards.**
2. **Keep your feet still and move your arm around and behind you. Stretch as far as you can and see exactly where you end up pointing to. Really stretch and remember the point.**
3. **Return your arm to the front and relax.**
4. **Close your eyes and be physically still, but in your imagination see yourself lifting the same arm and that now it is incredibly light and supple. Imagine that your whole body becomes light and supple as you see yourself moving your arm around and behind you. Imagine that you can move it so much further than before, and see in your mind's eye your arm moving beyond the previous point and**

glides freely further and further until it's almost all the way around, feeling so light and supple. Return your imaginary arm to the front and relax.

5. Now repeat the first step, really lifting your arm and pointing, and as you move it more freely now, stretch all the way around and notice how much further you can reach now.

If you visit www.powertochange.me.uk you can access a free audio download that will talk you through this technique.

Chances are that you can reach further the second time, sometimes much further. Why? What has changed? Your physical ability certainly hasn't changed; all that has happened is that you have experienced moving your arm further, so that goes into your memory as something you *can* do, as you have already done it! Then when you repeat the exercise, your mind draws on what it knows and replicates it. *It cannot differentiate between imagination and reality.*

Whether I am working with clients on a one-to-one basis, in a group workshop, or even training trainers and other therapists, I always teach them that your mind does not know the difference between an imagined thought and a real experience.

This can be used as both an advantage and a disadvantage. Have you ever been worried about someone; perhaps they are late coming home and you begin to imagine the worst, and as a result you experience real physical symptoms: elevated heart rate, sweating, all the usual 'fight or flight' responses? Then half an hour later they walk through the door and they are fine. You knew all along that they were probably safe, you had no evidence they were in any danger, yet in your imagination you created or imagined the worst possible outcome. Your mind *believed* the imagined scenario; that's why it evoked the stress response. If it had known you were only 'pretending' to worry, then it would not have sent any physical signals at all.

Conversely, if you really build something up in your mind and 'rehearse' how wonderful it will all be, and due to factors outside your control that doesn't happen, it is a much bigger disappointment than if you had just gone along with modest expectations. I remember when my children were much younger I planned a trip to Euro Disney the week before Christmas as their collective present, but I decided not to tell them as I wanted it to be a surprise. In my mind I imagined this fairytale holiday being totally idyllic. As it happened, my middle son was given a key role in the school Christmas play and wrote a 'Christmas rap' song to perform. Once I became aware of this I went in to school and told the teacher that he would be missing the last day of term, which was when the play was on, and that it was part of a big surprise. She agreed to let him carry on with the rehearsal, but to cover herself by having other children learning parts for the day. So there we sat the night before we went, the family all together, my perceived moment of bliss; I told them they could have their Christmas present early. This part, as you can imagine, went down well. I gave them the tickets for Euro Disney all wrapped up. So far so good – but when my son realized we were going the next morning he was absolutely mortified at the thought of missing the play and not performing his rap, and as a result there were tears and tantrums instead of my imagined joyful glee! When we got there it was raining, which continued the whole time we were there, and on the second day my daughter, who was about three years old at the time, got an upset tummy which meant she and I had to spend two days in our hotel room to be near the toilet, while the boys went to the park in the rain and got very wet. My disappointment was immense, and totally magnified because my expectations had been so high that I had already run the perfect holiday movie in my mind. This would not happen now, as I have the techniques and the understanding to prevent it, but at the time the reality was a crushing blow.

What you can learn from these examples is that if you worry about something that hasn't happened yet, and imagine that it will be awful, then you will experience it as awful even if it isn't; and if you build something up out of all practical expectations you are likely to be more disappointed than if you had had a more realistic approach.

The answer? Balance and a healthy dose of reality.

I have had people come to me for driving-test nerves. Perhaps they have failed once or twice. I always make it clear that I can remove the excess nervousness, but the reality is that no matter what I do, if they are not capable drivers they will not pass. In the same way I can work with actors for stage fright, and remove that, but they still need to learn their lines and their cues to give a great performance.

Great Expectations?

This chapter is really about understanding the way that you process information, and how that fits with your physical and environmental experiences. In a moment, I want you to put the book down and close your eyes for a moment or two, and reflect on how you think you process information, and if it serves you. Think about what your expectations are. Are you an optimist, ever seeing the glass as half-full? Or do you imagine the worst? What is your default setting for your imagination? Pause and close your eyes and reflect on this now.

Welcome back.

It is important to reflect on this, because if you want to change, then something you are doing now isn't working and it's helpful to find out what it is. If your computer had a problem with a specific programme, then your IT consultant would need to identify that specific problem and then delete and replace the damaged programme with an updated version. In most cases it's just one programme or fault that contaminates the whole computer, and once that's fixed the other programmes run smoothly. In the same way that anti-virus programmes can be installed to prevent future problems, then cb2 and tapping the side of your hand can work in exactly the same way and help detect and illuminate future problems.

Now let's learn some basic techniques that can replace the old, negative patterns or emotions with new, more empowering ones.

Anchoring

Anchoring is a basic technique that we all use every day, we just don't know it. Have you ever heard a piece of music on the radio that has taken you back to a specific time or place, or ever seen an image that reminded you of a certain event or location? The piece of music or image in these cases is, put simply, an *anchor*.

We create anchors all the time. Because the brain operates on a system of comparing present experiences with stored events, if it gets a 'match' then it accesses the previous file and opens it. For some it may be as simple as a word or phrase, for others a taste or smell. It can be literally anything.

I remember once walking through a shopping mall and literally bumping into an older gentleman, to the extent that I had to hold on to him to stop him from falling. As I did so I smelled his cologne, and in an instant I was taken back to being with my granddad, who used the same scent. It was as if the clock had stopped and time froze for a while, while I savoured the past experience. The whole event lasted only a few moments, maybe 20 or 30 seconds, but for ages afterwards I was thinking about my granddad and remembering him fondly. That was an anchor I didn't even know I had!

The important thing with anchoring is to create a *really* powerful, good anchor which you can literally bring to the surface whenever you need to remember to feel good. This is simple enough to do, but does require imagination.

Even if you can't create a good feeling, you can pretend, literally imagine, that you can feel good. Read through this exercise, then try it. The more you do it the better you will become at it, and the stronger your anchor will be. In later chapters we will be more specific with the anchors we set, but for now just learn to create a general 'feel good' anchor.

1. Sit back and close your eyes, and remember a time when you felt soooooo good. A time when you felt really happy. It doesn't matter how long ago, whom you were with, where you were or what has happened since, just isolate the feeling that you had. If you cannot access one, then think of a movie where you have seen a character feeling good, and really connect with that character and start to imagine how it feels to feel that good. If you are a visual thinker, make a picture and then make it bigger, brighter, bolder and more colourful. If you are an audio thinker, think about all you heard, qualify the sound and imagine it in the best-quality Dolby surround sound now. Think about where in your body you feel good, perhaps your chest, your tummy, perhaps your legs have gone weak! It doesn't matter where, but just notice how you are 'doing' feeling good.

2. Now take that feeling and imagine what it would be like if you doubled it. That's right, imagine you can feel twice as good. The feelings become even better, the pictures, the sounds and the emotions all work together to enhance your feelings and take you to another level of happiness.

3. Keep on doubling those good feelings until you are completely consumed by an overwhelming sense of feeling

good, and when you feel so good that you are physically beaming, squeeze the finger and thumb of your right hand together. Think of this as a 'save' button.

4. Clear your mind for a moment and think of blue bananas, then switch back very quickly to the REALLY good feeling and simultaneously squeeze the finger and thumb of your right hand together. Keep on doubling the feeling until you are once again overwhelmed with feeling good (even if it's pretend, go with it) and when you achieve that level, once more squeeze your right finger and thumb together.

5. Keep repeating Steps 3 and 4, generating overwhelming feelings of happiness and then switching to another thought and then back to the good feeling, each time squeezing that finger and thumb when you achieve the 'peak' of good feeling. Do this at least five or six times.

The finger-and-thumb squeeze becomes your 'anchor', working as a switch so that every time you squeeze them together your brain associates this with feeling happy.

The Swish

The Swish pattern is a really useful technique to learn and is really easy to do. It can be used to change any behaviour from smoking to not reacting in a certain way when something happens.

It can be done anytime, anywhere – and the more you do it, the better you get at it. Remember the brain learns quickly, so the Swish must be rapid and strong, and you have to *mean* it. Use your imagination so that you can create really vivid pictures.

There are two ways of creating pictures in your mind's eye; for this technique you will need to use both:

1. **You can be *associated*, which means seeing things through your eyes as if you are in the situation; literally imagining what you would be seeing. It's your internal representation of what you see.**
2. **You can be *disassociated*, which means creating an image of yourself that you can look at from an observer's perspective, just like looking at a picture or a movie.**

Before you begin, decide which behaviour you want to change, or Swish. As an example, let's say that something in your life acts as a trigger and makes you feel anxious, for example driving to work worrying about the day ahead. You will need to make two pictures: one of how you see things as you drive to work, and the second an image of you *without* this problem (how you would look if you had a positive feeling instead). Read through the following steps from start to finish before you begin, then do the exercise.

1. **Create the first picture, which is your 'cue' picture. That means what you see through your eyes, just before you start to feel anxious. Be *associated* – see it through your eyes. In our example this may be the dashboard of your car and the roads and signposts that tell you that you are on your way to work. If you were using this technique to change a behaviour such as smoking, it would be the sight of a cigarette just before it reaches your mouth. Spend some time looking at this picture and understanding 'how' you see it. Is it dark, bright, large, small? Identify the submodalities. Remove the image for a moment, but remember how to re-create or re-access it.**

2. **Now create an image of how you *want* to look and feel instead – perhaps confident and safe, in control perhaps or maybe just relaxed with the absence of any stress. With this image, be *disassociated*: see you how you would *like* to be. Make sure the image is so powerful that it creates within you a real desire to experience this for yourself. Look at how you see it: is it brighter, bigger, more colourful? Make sure you can really see it so clearly that you *want to have it.* Remove the image for a moment, but remember how to re-create or re-access it.**

3. **This time you are going to look at image 1 – that is, the behaviour you want to stop – but in the bottom left-hand corner of the image place a small box which is a collapsed view of the second, desired picture, much as you would see if you had minimized a file on your PC.**

4. Now *Swish* really fast – in less than a second, literally see the desired picture exploding onto the screen, completely annihilating the first picture. Make the swishing sound in your mind as you do this, and imagine feeling the different feelings you have as you see yourself set free of the problem. Let these good feelings sweep through your body in an instant. Imagine feeling so good as you see this image of you as you want to be.

Let the screen go blank, break your thought by thinking about baby green elephants, and then repeat stages 1 through 4 at least 5–10 times or until the first picture becomes so weak that when you try and see it, it automatically disappears to be replaced by the positive image – or perhaps you can no longer even see the first image and have already replaced it with the new image. Once you have done this successfully, hold that new image and anchor the feeling to the image.

If you visit www.powertochange.me.uk you can access a free audio download that will talk you through this technique.

Spinning

This is one of my favourite techniques, and it works particularly well after a TFT session (i.e. once the problem or issue has been removed). Often when you eliminate a problem, it leaves behind a kind of energy signature; although the problem has gone, there's a kind of benign feeling that sometimes remains as a result of having had it so long.

This exercise works best standing up; as with all exercises, read through the instructions carefully and step by step first, and then give it a try. In the context of this book we are working on the basis that you will have removed the problem first with TFT, but this exercise has great benefit in its own right even if you haven't. In this example, we will use a feeling of trauma, caused by a past event.

- **Stand up and think about where you felt the effects of the trauma in your body. Perhaps it was in your chest, perhaps it was a sick feeling in the pit of your gut? When you think about it, locate where specifically it is/was.**
- **Now think, if the trauma had a colour, what would it be?**
- **Now that you know exactly where in your body it is, and what colour it is, accept that it has energy and is a dynamic moving field.**
- **Now imagine a spinning wheel. This wheel spins the trauma into a thread, and when it spins 'in' the thread goes deeper inside your body, and when it spins 'out' the trauma is spun out of your body so that you will actually be able to see it in front of you. Make sure you can determine which**

direction of the wheel is 'in' and which is 'out'. This varies
from person to person and sometimes even from feeling to
feeling.

- Place one end of the thread on the spinning wheel and
  begin to spin the wheel outwards, in the direction that pulls
  the trauma *out* of your body; imagine the wheel turning
  faster and faster, as the thread is literally spun out of your
  body. Feel the pull of the thread as it spins faster and
  faster. Create a strong image in your mind's eye of exactly
  what it looks like as the trauma is moved outside of your
  body; notice the sound of the spinning wheel, perhaps a
  humming noise, or maybe it's a modern machine or an
  engine driving the wheel round. Sense the power of the
  wheel as you stand there. You are unable to prevent the
  wheel from spinning and spinning, and maybe the thread
  will begin to change colour or maybe it will just pull all the
  thread out until you notice the end of the thread spinning
  around in front of you on the wheel and you know it is all
  out.
- Even as the thread is removed, notice that the wheel keeps
  on turning and spinning, until after a few moments, it is
  spinning so fast that it shoots away out into the distance,
  like the Starship *Enterprise* going into warp drive. It's gone.
- Now, close your eyes for a moment and notice the empty
  space where it was. Maybe it's a large space, maybe not.
  Now is a good time to fill that space with something good.
  Use the happy thought you used earlier to anchor a good
  feeling, or choose another time or memory when you felt
  very safe and deeply happy. Spend some time imagining
  this, and then give it a colour.

- As you focus on this colour, imagine a ball of beautiful thread of this exact colour appearing in front of you on another spinning wheel, but this time it's turning in the opposite direction. Open yourself to receive this thread and begin to allow the spinning wheel to spin the new colour deep inside you to fill that gap. Notice how comfortable you are and how you can appreciate receiving that new feeling gratefully and graciously. There's nothing you can do but relax and receive it. Take all the time you need to enjoy the experience as the new feeling spins inside you, deeper and deeper. That's right. All the way in. Savour it.

- When you know that you have taken in more thread than you spun out, that you have an abundance of this new, good feeling, place your hand over the point where it entered your body and close it, for good. Seal the feeling in, and now imagine that feeling entering your bloodstream and flowing freely all through your body and into every cell, and deep within every cell into your DNA. Savour that process for as long as you want to.

You can use the action of placing your hand over your tummy (or wherever you spun the thread into) and the memory of the colour as a powerful anchor. Any time you need to feel good, simply do this and remember to remember how good it felt.

Timelines

There are many adaptations of working with 'time' in NLP. I love to use timelines. This simple technique can be adapted (as you will see in later chapters) for specific problems very effectively.

We all 'store' time around us spatially, within our field. The first time you think about this it can seem a bit strange, but trust me, it's important and very helpful to know where your 'timeline' is.

The following exercise will help you to locate yours. As always, read through all the instructions first, then go back to step one and do the exercise.

As this involves accessing lots of memories, establish that the only memories you are going to access for this are either happy, or benign. For example, remembering what your house looked like as a child, or even if you cleaned your teeth yesterday.

As I ask you to think about memories or events from your past, ask your unconscious mind to make you aware of where you 'feel' or 'see' them. Start by imagining you are standing on a dial, rather like a clock face but with no hands, so number 12 is directly ahead of you, number 3 to your right, 6 behind, 9 to your left and so on. Each time I ask you to access a memory, simply be aware of where it is placed. We are looking for a pattern or a line, although they do vary. For most people their memories will form a line (straight or wiggly) towards a specific number on the dial;

some may move upwards or downwards slightly as well, so just be aware of where specifically yours are in space.

Start with a recent memory of something that you did yesterday.

- **Now think of something that you did or that happened a few days or a week ago.**
- **Now think of something that you did or that happened a few weeks ago.**
- **Now think of something that you did or that happened a couple of months or so ago.**
- **Now think of something that you did or that happened about a year ago.**
- **Now think of something that you did or that happened about 2–3 years ago.**
- **Now think of something that you did or that happened about 7–8 years ago.**
- **Now think of something that you did or that happened about 10–15 years ago.**
- **Now think of something that you did or that happened about 20 or more years ago.**
- **Now think of something that you did or that happened when you were a young child, perhaps a school memory.**
- **Now think of your earliest happy memory.**

Using your dominant arm, point to where in space you see, feel or sense that these memories are. Remember that point, and lower your arm.

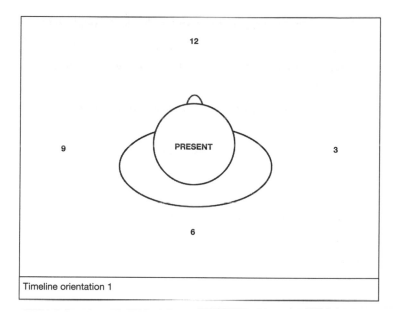

Timeline orientation 1

Now think about your future. You get to play a little here, as you can create an imaginary future based on what you would like to happen, and it will work, even though it is a 'created' memory.

- **Imagine something you know or would like to happen tomorrow.**
- **Imagine something you know or would like to happen next week.**
- **Imagine something you know or would like to happen in a month or so.**
- **Imagine something you know or would like to happen in 6 months or so.**
- **Imagine something you know or would like to happen in a year or so.**

- **Imagine something you know or would like to happen in 2–3 years.**
- **Imagine something you know or would like to happen in 5–7 years.**
- **Imagine something you know or would like to happen in 12–15 years.**
- **Imagine something you know or would like to happen in 20 years.**
- **Imagine something you know or would like to happen as far as you want to see right now into your future.**

Using your other arm, point to where in space you see, feel or sense the 'future memories' are.

Using the figure below, draw a line outwards in the direction of your past and a line in the direction of your future.

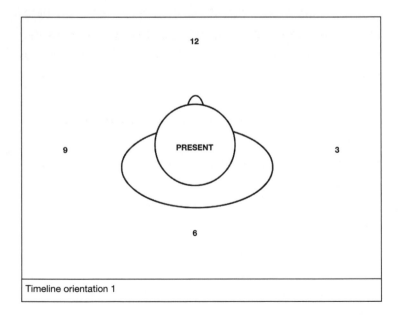

Timeline orientation 1

Now look at where you *store* time. There are lots of theories as to the various directions, but in my experience the best place for your past is *behind* you. And the best place for your future is *straight in front of* you. If you are not in this alignment, then do the following exercise:

Close your eyes and visualize your past timeline. See it as a rope, string, thread, pole, whatever works for you, but notice its place in space and its colour. Now imagine a safe pair of hands, or some invisible good energy, gently but firmly taking your past timeline and putting it *behind* you. Take all the time you need to do this properly. When you know your past has been placed behind you, is stretched out horizontally in chronological order as it happened, anchor it there and accept its new position. Say thank you. You may or may not notice a change in its colour. It doesn't matter, it's behind you now, for good.

Now visualize your future, and in exactly the same way move it and place it directly in front of you, and as you do so lengthen it and fire it out into the future so far that you cannot see the end of it. It's a beautiful, infinite horizontal line that you can see clearly. This line represents infinite possibilities.

Now complete the following diagram as to where your new timeline is located.

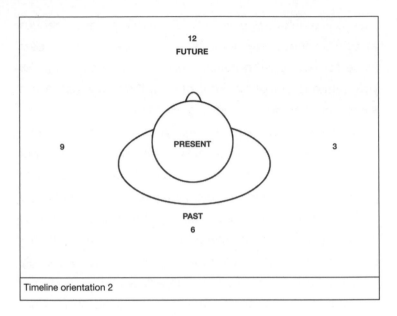

12
FUTURE

9

PRESENT

3

PAST
6

Timeline orientation 2

If your past was in your forward vision, or even your peripheral vision, no doubt you were living in the past to some extent, and some traumas or past experiences were still affecting you and holding you back, maybe stopping you from seeing your future clearly. If this is you then this exercise is especially important.

We'll be taking a look at how to refine this even further in a later chapter.

Your Internal Dialogue

Be careful what you say – you might be listening!

We all have it, whatever you call it – internal chatter, inner voice, internal dialogue – it's within all of us. It is like a running commentary on life and can be heard in the form of reminders, comments on your surroundings, thoughts abut yourself or others. It's probably the most influential part of our make-up. How often have you 'heard' yourself say, 'You can't do that!' and believed it? How often do you accept the negative chatter without even questioning it? Even worse, how often do you let your internal voice insult you, using language you would never accept from anyone else?

As a therapist, when I am working with someone with low self-esteem and I ask them what is the worst thing they ever say to themselves, some of the replies I get are hideously offensive. When I then ask if they would say this to anyone else they know, perhaps a friend, the answer is a resounding 'No!' So why is it that some people allow their negative chatter to be so destructive? My experience tells me that people just don't know how to turn it off, or change it.

Try this very simple exercise: close your eyes to cut out all visual signals, and focus on the voice in your head. Have it count to 10. Now have it count to 10 and miss out the number 5. Now have it count to 10 in a very sexy French accent, still missing out the number 5. You can do it, can't you?

What you have just done is to demonstrate very clearly to yourself that *you* are in control of your inner voice. The problem occurs when the 'default setting' is *negative*. Who wouldn't be influenced by negative, insulting comments being fired at them all day long?

I remember one day in particular when I was training with Richard Bandler. As with many training sessions, there were a lot of 'course junkies' there. I mean this as an observation with no offence intended, but you do find a lot of people just going from course to course and never actually putting what they learn into practice, always believing they need to do just one more course to become good enough. Often these are the people who sit at the front taking copious notes, completely in a trance the whole time, often starstruck by the presenter.

Richard Bandler is an expert at 'reading' a group, and on this particular day there were upwards of 500 people in the room, and he was chatting about our inner voice and internal dialogue and how it influences us. He has a very hypnotic style and language pattern in any event, but during this particular session, even more than usual, people were dropping into a deep, eyes-open trance all around the room; they were literally hanging on to his every word. When he was asking questions such as, 'How do you feel when your inner voice says something rude and offensive?' and getting agreement from the group about how bad this was and how great it would be if it were possible to do something to stop it, heads were nodding and people were moving forwards in their chairs, straining to hear the next piece of information. He began to suggest that there *was* something you could do to stop it – again people slid forwards in their chairs in almost frenzied anticipation of the next technique.

Master of the build-up, Bandler then asked us to allow our negative commentary to insult us in the worst way possible, and really get in touch with how that made us feel. From the stage he encouraged us all to turn up the volume and listen to it profoundly; as he did so he said, 'In a moment I am going to show you how to turn it off.' A palpable blend of fear and excitement filled the room, as all these people, some head in hands, were reacting simultaneously to their internal negative voice but also to the prospect of finding a way to stop it. Richard allowed this to go on for some time until he said, 'Now I want you to go inside your mind and say the following to that internal voice ... ' Silence filled the room and the anticipation reached fever pitch as we all 'went inside', poised to repeat this wonderful new technique we were about to learn ... from the stage Richard boomed out into the microphone, 'TELL IT TO SHUT THE FUCK UP!'

Five hundred sharp intakes of breath later – there was a stunned silence followed by a few giggles. Then Richard asked, 'Anyone still got their negative chatter?' Not one arm was raised. I was at the back of the room laughing out loud thinking what a great trick it was! I learned so much that day just watching other people, it was fantastic.

This technique works because it does two things: first, it breaks your pattern; it takes you from feeling hurt and dejected and 'doing' sad, to suddenly thinking 'Who is this rude man on the stage?' Breaking a state or breaking a pattern is critical, and an essential technique to learn. I bet many of you have done this automatically for friends to get them out of a bad/sad mood. If you are sitting moping about something, playing it over and over again, feeling worse and worse, and a friend comes along and says 'That's enough of that, I am taking you out!', then it breaks your state. In order to feel sad you have to 'do' sad. You have to run that internal voice, probably along with some nice negative pictures, on a nice long loop. If you do that you can get really good at feeling bad. I have worked with people who could have a PhD in feeling sad, they had become so expert at 'doing' it. What is sad is that it doesn't change anything, in fact it closes off doorways of opportunity that might have otherwise opened.

The second thing is, when you say something as if you mean it, it has an effect. When Richard boomed out his obscenity from the stage, he really meant it – trust me, he was completely convincing!

In the same way that we store pictures and even time spatially, we also have a spatial location for various internal auditory sounds and voices. Try this exercise. As before, read it through first, then do it:

Allow yourself to hear your negative commentary (if you have one) or think of an insulting remark that someone has said to you that has affected you.

Now allow yourself to notice where specifically it is coming from. Is it behind you, directly into your left ear, your right ear, is the voice right in front of you? Notice where it is. Notice also how it makes you feel, and where in your body you are feeling it.

Now think about a cartoon character or any TV or movie character that has a funny voice. It might be Daffy Duck, Scooby Doo, Mickey Mouse, it doesn't matter which one it is as long as it makes you laugh or smile when you think of it. Have it say a short sentence directly to you, for example mine would be Scooby Doo saying, ' Helloooooooooo Janet, this is Scooby dooby dooby Dooooooooooo asking how are yooooooooou?' with perhaps even the Scooby Doo music in the background. Do it now, and allow yourself to notice where specifically this voice is coming from. Is it behind you, directly into your left ear, your right ear, is the voice right in front of you? Notice where it is. Notice also how it makes you feel, and where in your body you are feeling it. How is this different to the first voice?

Now use the vocabulary from the first voice, your negative chatter, and have your cartoon character say those exact same words. Repeat it a few times and notice where the sound is coming from and how it makes you feel.

Chances are that when you take the time to do this exercise properly, you'll notice it's *not* the words that you use that are offensive, it's the *way* you say them. You are too convincing with your negative voice! But when your comedy voice says this same stuff, you almost laugh at it; it's completely unbelievable; it just does not have the same effect. What this means is that words only have the meaning that *you* give them, and this is determined by the way in which you hear or receive them. So when you change the way you speak to yourself *and* what you say, the effects can be quite dramatic.

If you want to be good at something, then start telling yourself you *are* good at it *now*. Of course you will still have to learn the techniques, but you have to believe and convince yourself that you can do this. Create a statement or affirmation that defines specifically who you are and how you want to live your life. Every morning when you are in the bathroom take a look in the mirror and say your statement out loud – send it out there into the universe and you may be amazed at how quickly it comes back to you. We will talk more about this in later chapters.

NLP is, in essence, all about attitude and choice. I love TFT; every day, whether working with clients on a one-to-one basis or in a seminar or bootcamp, I use and teach it to astonishingly good effect. What makes it even better is that, when combined with the NLP techniques I have shown you here, it's possible not only to eliminate negative thoughts, emotions and feelings (even those brought about by the most horrid events) but also to create a completely new set of skills and ways of processing information that gives you a wealth of new possibilities and options, so that you can live the life you were truly born to live. No one was ever born to suffer, and that includes you.

Your Emotional Toolkit

If you have a specific problem, the information in the chapters that follow is designed to be used for self-treatment, and is based on everything you have already learned from this book. You may have already noticed a significant improvement in how you feel just from reading this far; in any event, simply choose the chapter that is most relevant for you and work through the individual exercises. Keep the book as a future reference and as an emotional toolkit.

Each chapter from here on in is effectively a 'stand alone' chapter – that is, you do not need to read about how to eliminate a phobia if your problem is anxiety; simply go to the chapter about eliminating anxiety and work through that. You may, however, need to use other chapters at a later stage or to help someone else, so the book is a great resource to keep.

In each chapter there is some repetition of what you have already learned; this is for your convenience so that you don't have to go back to earlier chapters each time you come to do an exercise or treatment.

Intent

Whichever of the following chapters is the right one for you, approach it with an open mind and *intent* to get a great result. In therapy I have found that having the right *intent* when using any of the techniques I have shown you is vital for the successful outcome. The power of your belief is immense, so you can believe now that you can use these techniques effectively and for your highest good.

I would like you to take a moment now and read the following excerpt from *Meditations and Inspirations* by Virginia Satir. You can do the mediation as you read; there's no need to be lying down with your eyes closed in order to achieve the desired result. You can reflect on what you read as you read it, and achieve a great result.

'Begin now to be in touch with your breathing.
Adjust your body so it feels comfortable. Let yourself
become prepared. Ask the part of yourself that takes
in information and new experiences to allow you to be

relaxed and open. Remember as you hear and see, to let things come in. Taste them and allow them to be swallowed when your inside says they fit.

'At this moment, could you allow yourself to remember that you have lived successfully so far? The way is open for you to add to yourself. Could you allow yourself to be aware that there is so much about a human being, and about human beings being together on this planet in the universe, from which we learn?

'We can learn what we need in abundance, and to be happy, productive, respected human beings. That we may not be fully there, does not mean we don't have the ability, only that we haven't found it and learned how to use it yet. Everyone has this human potential.

'Give a message of love to your left brain. Make it a strong message of love, because your left hemisphere doesn't know yet that your right hemisphere will help you in your learnings.

'Allow yourself now, with your eyes open, to feel that body of yours – that gorgeous temple, that magnificent miracle. Ease into your seat in a balanced way, making sure both feet are on the floor. If there are any little tight places as you take in your breath, send the breath through your body. Stop to smile when you find a tight place and let the tensions leave on an outgoing breath.

'Notice that, whether you are aware of it or not, your breath is coming and going. As you sit there, getting ready for some new learning, you may want to give your breath an inspiring colour. This colour could then move

to all parts of your body, filling it. Smiling as it goes in, this colour fills and nurtures you.

'Let yourself come in touch with your breathing, and feel your self-nurturing through your breath ...

'Now go to that place deep inside yourself and give yourself a message of appreciation. Maybe now you can give yourself permission to let go of all those things you have carried around that are no longer of use. Bid them a fond farewell. Let them go, and be in touch with things you have that fit you well right now. Give yourself permission to add that which you need.

'With your message of appreciation to yourself, you can now be ready for whatever you are going to learn today.'
Virginia Satir

Part 4
Putting TFT into Action

Eliminating Phobias

According to the American Psychiatric Association, a phobia is 'an irrational or excessive fear of an object or situation which in most cases involves a sense of endangerment or harm'. Phobias are characterized by an excessive fear, out of all proportion to the situation or object.

If you are suffering from a phobia, then you may recognize some of the following physical symptoms:

- **nausea or vomiting**
- **breathlessness**
- **dizziness**
- **tight chest**
- **rapid heart rate**
- **elevated blood pressure**
- **temporary paralysis**
- **inability to function generally.**

The extent to which you suffer these physical symptoms depends, of course, on the severity of the phobia. Even a minor physical response can be quite debilitating and restricting. Most people with phobias do recognize the fear as irrational, but believe that by keeping it they are keeping themselves safe. I know someone who has a shark phobia (who hasn't?!) and as a result will not swim in the sea. I have offered to eliminate it for her, but she will not even consider it as she believes her phobia keeps her safe by stopping her swimming in the sea. Logically, even without this phobia, you would not deliberately swim in shark-infested waters. You must trust your natural instincts to keep you safe, these are in no way inhibited by removing your phobia; for example, if you rid yourself of a fear of heights, this doesn't mean you are going to the top of a tall building to jump off because you have no fear any more.

Eliminating your phobia in no way *inhibits your natural survival instincts or your ability to react to certain situations and to keep yourself safe.*

Over the years I have had many people come to me with unusual phobias, everything from a fear of butterflies or balloons to baked beans. Here are some of the most common phobias:

Arachnophobia	Fear of spiders
Social phobia	Fear of public speaking and perceived negative feedback
Aerophobia (also known as Aviaphobia)	Fear of flying
Agoraphobia	Fear of not being able to escape, can be open spaces or crowded places
Claustrophobia	Fear of enclosed spaces
Acrophobia	Fear of heights
Emetophobia	Fear of vomit
Brontophobia	Fear of thunderstorms
Necrophobia	Fear of dead things
Mysophobia	Fear of germs

The only fear we are born with is the natural fear of heights. As we grow older and we learn about our environment and how to keep ourselves safe, this fear subsides; when someone has acrophobia then the normal process of learning has not taken place and the fear of heights remains. All other phobias are the result of experiences and are 'learned'. It may not even be your own individual experience that has caused your phobia. Let me give you an example.

I had a client with a frog phobia that was so chronic that she could barely go outside the house during certain months of the year. After I chatted to her for a while to elicit when the phobia had begun and how she had 'learned' to be phobic, she told me she had never personally had a bad experience with frogs, but that her mother had had such an extreme frog phobia that no images or pictures of frogs were allowed in the house, to the extent that all of the encyclopaedias and books in the house had to be vetted and any pictures of frogs cut out. Apparently her mother would not be able to sleep if she thought there was even a picture of a frog in the house. If they were out anywhere where there might be a frog, her mother was prone to anxiety attacks. As a result, my client learned from a very early age to be phobic.

After the first session I took her outside in the garden, and on a warm dusky evening she looked in the pond to try and find frogspawn or a frog. While she didn't enjoy this process, she was able to do it without a phobic reaction. After the second session she sent me a lovely email saying she had bought a soft toy frog for her bedroom and a fridge magnet frog.

If you want to see the power of TFT in action, you can watch a clip of me eliminating a chronic needle phobia on my website www.powertochange.me.uk. And now, in this chapter, you will learn how to eliminate a phobia yourself.

What Can You Expect After You Have Eliminated Your Phobia?

It is important to understand fully the likely outcome after treatment. If you are treating yourself for a dog phobia, for example, then it would not be wise, even for the most discerning dog lover, to approach any and every dog for a cuddle. In other words, eliminating your phobia does not mean you suddenly love all dogs; in fact you may still really dislike them. What it *does* mean is that you'll be able to look at a dog, acknowledge you don't like it very much, but *not* have a phobic reaction or any physiological response to it. It's no different to seeing anything else you don't like.

I used to have a mild flying phobia; I have now eliminated it but I still don't like flying. But I don't like gooseberries, either; it's no big deal. The only difference is that avoiding gooseberries does not prevent me from travelling, so I don't have to put myself in a situation where I'd *have* to eat them. If I had to eat gooseberries in order to get to Australia, though, then I certainly would.

I once treated a spider phobic who had been known to call a friend in the middle of the night when she found a spider in her bath, and her friend would have to come over and remove the spider before my client would go back in the house. She had a violent reaction even to looking at one sealed in a jar. When I finished the treatment she could (after we let it out on her carpet – purely for television purposes!) place a cup over it, slide a piece of paper under it and take it outside to let it go and watch it scamper away. No more phobia. A week or so later she emailed me to say the phobia hadn't gone, and that she had found a spider in the bath the previous night, put a cup over it and taken it outside, and the spider was 'horrible'. This is not a phobia; this is just someone who does not like spiders. When I asked her if she could have got the spider out of the house herself before the treatment, she said absolutely not! The phobia was gone; what she was left with was a dislike of spiders.

So – start with the end in mind. You can eliminate your phobia, so that in that specific situation you can (if you choose) maintain a healthy dislike for whatever it is, but you will not have a phobic reaction. After a while you may even forget that you don't like it and actually become more and more tolerant of it.

Seven Steps

Follow these next seven steps carefully, referring back to earlier chapters if you need to. Make sure you are somewhere quiet where you can concentrate and focus totally on what you are doing. Think of this as a proper treatment or therapy session. I would not treat you in a snatched 5 minutes between tasks, so allow yourself time to do this properly for yourself. It may take anything from 20 minutes to an hour, and you may wish to repeat all seven steps another time to reinforce all you have changed. Take as much time as you need, as often as you need.

It is important that you are in a space where you feel safe and secure. You may need to have access to something such as a laptop so you can access pictures or movies if you need something to help you to get in the thought field, as explained earlier.

The order of these steps is important; as I have explained, the most thorough approach is to go back into the past and remove the *cause* of the phobia *before* you remove the actual phobia, then eliminate the *current* fear, then eliminate any *future* fear. We will be using primarily TFT, but also an effective NLP treatment to complete the process.

Now go to that place deep inside yourself and give yourself a message of appreciation. Maybe now you can give yourself permission to let go of all those things you have carried around with you that are no longer of use. Bid them a fond farewell. Let them go, and be in touch with things you have that fit you well right now. Give yourself permission to add that which you need.

> 'With your message of appreciation to yourself, you can now be ready for whatever you are going to learn today.'
> **Virginia Satir**

Steps 1–4

Steps 1–4 are about taking an accurate history of the problem right up to the current day. This is exactly what I would do if I were treating you. Complete all the stages, allowing yourself, if necessary, to close your eyes and take a moment or two to go 'inside' and really feel the emotions.

Step 1: Identify the Phobia

It sounds obvious, but make sure you know *specifically* what you are dealing with: for example, 'a fear of animals' is too vague; think about which animal, specifically, you are most afraid of. You may need to 'chunk down' from a generic fear to that of which you are most afraid.

Write down your phobia.

When you think about your phobia, what is the SUD (between 1 and 10)? Write that down, too.

Step 2a: Think about the First Time You Had this Phobic Reaction

Go back to *before* you had your phobia, then to the exact time when you learned to be phobic. What happened to teach you that response? I have known a chronic snake phobia occur after a woman's brother threw a plastic snake at her when she was about 10 years old; as she screamed and threw her arms up into the air, it moved and fell into her lap. The result was a phobic reaction, even though she had never actually seen a real snake other than on TV.

Write down the time or event – remember exactly what happened. Take an SUD reading and write that down, too.

Step 2b: Think about Exactly How that First Reaction Made You Feel

Of course there was fear, but what else? Was there anger or rage? Was there embarrassment or shame?

Write down your specific feelings.

Step 3: Think about Later Times or Events When You've Felt Traumatized by the Phobia

If there are no more times other than the initial trigger event, move on to Step 4. Chronology is *not* important, just write them down in the order of severity and give each an SUD of 1–10.

Step 4: Think about Your Fear *Now*

Put yourself (use props or images if necessary) in the situation as best as possible and take an SUD reading. Write it down.

The Basic Treatment

Now you have an accurate history, the treatment can begin.

Go back to steps 2a and 2b and look at the emotions involved in your experience, and select the most appropriate sequence from those shown below.

If the following treatment sequences do not work fully for you, and you have tried all the corrective treatments, then go to the table on page 107 and select a more appropriate algorithm based on your feelings.

I will guide you through a basic treatment here, but if you need a more detailed reminder, do revisit the earlier section on TFT protocol.

Basic trauma and fear

eb   e   a   c   9g   sq

Trauma with rage

eb   e   a   c   oe   c   9g   sq

or

eb   oe   e   a   c   9g   sq

Trauma with anger

eb   e   a   c   tf   9g   sq

or

eb   tf   e   a   c   9g   sq

Trauma with embarrassment or shame

eb e   a   c   un   ul   c   9g   sq

Having chosen the right sequence for you, tune in to the exact thought field, and think about the first event or trauma that was the cause or the beginning of your phobia. For this example I will use the basic trauma algorithm, but if you want to select one of the others, simply use that sequence instead.

The Rules

1. Tune in to the thought field and check the SUD. If it's different from before, write it down.
2. Treat as if there were a reversal and tap the side of your hand (**sh**) and under your nose (**un**) 20 times; then tap the sequence eb e   a   c
3. Take an SUD. If it is going down, then continue to Step 4; if not, complete the corrective treatment (*see* page 60) and then repeat Step 2.
4. Do the 9 gamut sequence:

   * Tap the gamut spot continually; at the same time:
   * Close your eyes/open your eyes (long blink)
   * Keep your head still and, moving your eyes only, look down to one side (R) and back to centre.
   * Look down to the other side (L) and back to centre.
   * Look down as if you were looking at number 6 on a clock dial, then move your eyes round to 9 o'clock, then 12 o'clock, 3 o'clock, and all the way round in a circle as if you were looking at every number on the dial, finishing back at number 6.
   * Now repeat the full circle but in the other direction.

- Hum a few notes (e.g. the musical scales or 'happy birthday') out loud.
- Count out loud 1-2-3-4-5.
- Hum out loud again.

5. Repeat the sequence eb e a c
6. Take an SUD. If it is going down, then repeat Steps 1–5 until the SUD is 2 or less. If it is not going down, then complete the corrective treatment on page 60, and then repeat Step 5.
7. When the SUD is a 2 or less, do the eye roll:
   - Tap the gamut spot continually for at least 30 taps and, keeping your head still, look as far down as you can. Keep tapping and gradually move your eyes forwards and upwards until you are looking right up into your eyebrows.

Corrective Treatment

If there is no reduction in SUD, then one of four things is happening:

1. You are not in the thought field.
2. You are using the wrong sequence.
3. You are in psychological reversal (PR).
4. You have toxins (IETs) present.

Check the first two, then correct for PR:

Try the first point of the corrective treatment (tapping the side of your hand). You will only need to use the others if this does not work. For more detailed information on corrective treatments, refer back to page 60.

- Tap the side of your hand 20+ times (karate spot). This is known as PR1.
- Run your fingers along the underside of your LEFT collarbone from the shoulder to the centre of your chest. If you find a spot that is sore, then gently but firmly rub this spot using circular motions towards the centre of your chest, until the soreness subsides.
- Tap under your nose 20+ times. This is known as PR2.
- Do collarbone breathing (*see* page 62).

When you can think about the past event with a negligible response, move on to Step 3. This is your list of all the other times when you have been traumatized by this phobia. If there aren't any, other than the initial event, then move on to Step 4.

As mentioned earlier, dealing with any emotion can be like peeling an onion, and it's important to eliminate each and every layer. Do not be lazy here; do it properly and systematically. Use exactly the same protocol as I have just shown you for the initial trauma – that is, identify the emotions, select the algorithm, take an SUD and follow the same procedure detailed above. You will need to write down the information for each 'layer'; this will help you to focus and get in the thought field. You must also make a note of the SUD *before* you start.

Remember, this is *not* about recollecting chronologically; go in order of the most severe or traumatic event. Anything above a 3 on the SUD scale should be treated.

When you have completed treating your past events, move on to Step 4: how you feel *now*. You may or may not find that, as a result of clearing past traumas, the SUD has already reduced. Take a moment, use props if necessary, and really go 'inside' and think about what specifically is the worst part of your phobia. It's important to chunk down here; for example if you have a phobia about flying you will need to go through the whole process of flying and everything that's involved, starting with the check-in, going through security, boarding the plane, watching the in-flight demo, when the doors shut, etc. There may be a collection of 'triggers' or it may be just one. If you are working on a fear of thunder, for instance, you may or may not visualize lightning with it, it may be worse in the daytime or the night-time, or if you are alone. Start with the very worst scenario and take an SUD, and treat that first. Write down all the triggers and their specific SUD, then work through them one by one. You may notice that, as you eliminate some, others are automatically reduced or disappear as well.

The general anxiety/fear algorithm is

e   a   c   9g   sq

If you have a more complex emotion than simple fear, you may want to use one of the following sequences – or one of the ones on page 107, if it seems more accurately to describe your emotional state:

Basic anxiety and fear

e   a   c   9g   sq

Anxiety with rage

e   a   c   oe   9g   sq

_**or**_

e   oe   a   c   9g   sq

Anxiety with anger

e   a   c   tf   9g   sq

_**or**_

e   tf   e   a   c   9g   sq

Anxiety with embarrassment or shame

e   a   c   un   ul   c   9g   sq

Using Rules 1–7 on page 173, carry out treatments for all necessary trigger points and current fears, until all aspects of the problem, when you think about them now, generate an SUD of 2 or less.

You can now move on to the next stage of treatment.

Step 5: Future Time

You may have cleared the phobia _now_, and there's a good chance the phobia is gone for good, but let's make sure you have also eliminated it from your _future_, so that if at any time you are faced with your old phobia you know it has gone. To do this your thoughts have to be projected into a future time.

- **Picture in your mind's eye being in that phobic situation sometime in the future, perhaps even 12 months from now. If you have anything that registers as a 3 or more on the SUD scale, write it down.**
- **Choose the most appropriate anxiety algorithm sequence and follow Rules 1–7 (on page 173) until the SUD is a 2**

or less. As before, this may or may not be like peeling an onion and may only involve one situation, or several. **Be thorough.**

- **Check your work: imagine any and all situations where you may be faced with your old phobia. Remember, if you are in a phobic situation and any level of anxiety surfaces, you can immediately and on the spot use the anxiety algorithm to clear it.**

Sometimes it's just not possible to get totally in the thought field just using your imagination or YouTube. Flying is a good example. Normally I can eliminate any trace of a fear of flying in my treatment room, but when the client is actually next on a plane he achieves a state he just could not access in the comfort of a therapy session. This is why it is important to learn the basic anxiety algorithm and the PR corrections so that you can, if you need to, 'top up' your treatment any time. Some public speakers and actors I have worked with use the anxiety sequence before any and every performance, as each one is a completely new experience in its own right. Just knowing you have a great resource, quite literally at your fingertips, is very reassuring.

A number of years ago (before I had the psychological techniques I have now!) I had a chronic back condition which resulted in major surgery in the form of a spinal fusion, taking bone from my hip and fusing it into my spine. I was in a lot of pain and at the same time had two young children to look after, and life was very tough. I became very stressed physically and emotionally and couldn't sleep. After a few weeks I went to the GP, who gave me sleeping tablets. That night I put them by the bed and thought to myself, 'I will see how I go without them, but if I need them I know they are there.' Any anxiety about not sleeping vanished and I slept like a log, with no tablets. What the tablets did was give me a sense of reassurance, a resource that I could use if I needed it. Knowing how to use TFT is the same: if you are ever faced with a phobic situation, you know you have your medication (in the form of TFT) right at your fingertips.

Note: For most phobias the basic anxiety algorithm **e a c 9g sq** is appropriate, but please note that for turbulence while flying, or moving spiders, for example, the sequence is **a e c 9g sq**, as shown in the table on page 107.

If you have completed all the steps correctly, chances are that you have no more phobia. However, if it remains at all, or in part, then use the following techniques to eliminate it completely.

If you have noticed no reduction at all using TFT, then you may need to seek out a TFT Diagnostic or VT therapist who can diagnose you for any IETs (toxins, *see* page 96).

Make sure that you use collarbone breathing morning and night (page 62) as part of your daily routine, and tap the side of your hand regularly throughout the day in order to keep yourself out of PR.

Step 6: Fast Phobia Cure
This is one of the earliest NLP techniques and can work very well either in its own right or as a complement to TFT. It takes 5 or 10 minutes to do, depending how many times you need to repeat the exercise, and works particularly well for visual (right-brain) thinkers. Make sure you are sitting comfortably

and can relax so that you can focus your mind. Before you start: take an SUD.

Imagine you are walking into an empty cinema. Choose the chair right in the centre of the front row and sit down and look at the blank screen.

Leave your body there and imagine that you can float up out of your body and behind it, all the way back into the projection room so that you can see yourself sitting there in the front row, and look at yourself looking at the blank screen.

Think about your phobia, capture the moment the phobia would begin and freeze-frame it, see it as a still picture and put that image on the screen in colour. This is you a split second before you had the phobic response.

Run the complete movie of your phobia, from your safe vantage position in the projection room, and watch yourself watching the movie all the way to the end, to the point where it's over and you can see you are safe. Freeze-frame this safe image at the end of the movie and make it black and white.

Now float back down into your body and watch the movie again, this time as if it was filmed through your eyes.

At the end of the movie make the last image still and black and white again, and step into the image and be fully associated, seeing what you would see through your eyes, and feel how you feel. Now play the movie backwards, very quickly, still in black and white, and add a silly cartoon-type soundtrack (This may look and sound rather like a Charlie Chaplin movie effect, and that's fine). At the end of the movie freeze-frame the beginning picture (as it was originally, only now it's black and white).

Now, very quickly, imagine the screen goes completely white.

Step out of the blank screen and sit down in your chair looking at your white screen.

Test yourself and see if the SUD has been reduced. If it is more than a 2, repeat the process until there is no phobic response at all.

You may want to use some of the other techniques such as the Swish or Spinning, described earlier, to reinforce all that you have changed. In particular, set yourself a very strong *anchor* to a time when you have felt really safe:

1. **Sit back and close your eyes, and remember a time when you felt totally safe. It doesn't matter how long ago, whom you were with, where you were or what has happened since, just isolate the feeling that you had. If you cannot remember a time, then simply imagine how it will feel to be totally safe. If you are a visual thinker, make a picture and then make it bigger, brighter, bolder and more colourful. If you are an audio thinker, think about all you heard, qualify the sound and imagine it in the best-quality Dolby surround sound now. Think about where in your body you feel safe, perhaps your chest, your tummy; just notice how you are 'doing' feeling safe.**

2. Now take that feeling of safety and imagine what it would be like if you doubled it. That's right, imagine you can feel twice as safe. The feelings become even better, the pictures, the sounds and the emotions all work together to enhance your feelings and take you to another level of safety.

3. Keep on doubling those good feelings until you are completely consumed by an overwhelming sense of feeling safe, and when you feel so good and safe that you are physically beaming, squeeze the finger and thumb of your right hand together. Think of this as a 'save' button.

4. Clear your mind for a moment and think of blue bananas, then switch back very quickly to the REALLY good feeling and simultaneously squeeze the finger and thumb of your right hand together. Keep on doubling the good feelings until you are once again overwhelmed with feeling good (even if it's pretend, go with it), and when you achieve that level once more, squeeze your right finger and thumb together.

5. Keep repeating steps 3 and 4, using the thumb-squeeze to generate the overwhelming feelings of safety happiness and then switching to another thought and then back to the good feeling, each time squeezing that finger and thumb to act as a switch to access the 'peak' of feeling good. Do this at least five or six times.

The finger-and-thumb squeeze becomes your 'anchor', working as a switch, so that every time you squeeze them together your brain associates this with feeling happy and safe.

What Happens Now?

Now you have eliminated your phobia you should be able to face the previously anxiety-provoking situation with a complete absence of fear. It doesn't mean you will now *like* the situation (although you might!), but with the phobia gone you can feel in control of yourself again. Make sure you learn the basic PR corrections and also the anxiety algorithm so that you have all the tools you need, should you experience a recurrence or any similar emotion.

>>>Case Study: Kerry

As I've already mentioned, some time ago I did some work for Central ITV where we asked viewers to contact me with their problems and I would 'change their lives'. We were inundated with many applications, but more that anything else there were phobias. I would like to tell you about one in particular whom we chose to film.

Kerry had a chronic needle phobia, she was heavily pregnant and also already had a young child who needed immunizing. She was absolutely terrified. When we arrived with the cameras she was a little anxious about what the treatment might involve, and her mum and husband were on hand to tell us just how debilitating Kerry's phobia could be. The presenter, Alison, had brought along some sterilized needles so we could mimic the injection in order to get Kerry into the thought field. As soon as Kerry saw these she ran to the toilet and locked herself in, crying uncontrollably. The camera crew were trying to calm her down but I was just keen to start tapping. We persuaded Kerry to come out and I tapped the sequence. Within one minute her breathing had calmed and she'd stopped

183

crying; within 5 minutes all trace of the phobia was gone. I did some other exercises and visualizations with Kerry as well (not least because we had several more minutes of airtime to fill!), but in essence TFT alone had 'collapsed' her phobia, literally in minutes. Don't take my word for it – check it out for yourself at www. powertochange.me.uk

>>>Testimonial: Terry – Public Speaking Phobia

Dear Janet, I wanted to give you an update since you treated me for my public speaking phobia; yesterday I was 'forced' to give an hour-long detailed presentation on stage in front of 100 people, all of whom were 'technical'. The week building up to this was not comfortable and I had to represent several technology departments from my team, presenting information I understand but am not an expert in. For some strange reason (or perhaps not so strange) I walked calmly up and gave an hour-long technical presentation without a hitch. Afterwards lots of people gave me extremely good and positive feedback. For those who also know me and my previous 'condition', they said they'd noticed a vast change for the better. They said it was as if I had been doing this for a long time, no nerves at all and full of confidence and in complete control. I even dropped in a few lines that made everyone (including me!) laugh.

The accounts director was also there, and made a point of talking to me afterwards, saying it was good to see confidence, vision and long-term strategy within the account. He thanked me for the presentation and for making him feel better about delivering the £20-million contract we won last week. (This guy has a fearsome reputation and usually is one to be avoided.)

Anyway, clearly subconsciously something has happened, and I wish to say a big thank you! In fact, in all honesty, I enjoyed it!

I really, really want to say thank you. This issue has held me back for years, but not any more, I have another big presentation next week and I am not even thinking about it!

>>>Testimonial: Eileen – Claustrophobia and Fear of Flying

If I think back to my youth, I can recall isolated incidents of claustrophobia, but from 2002 the incidents got closer together. The 'attacks' were very real: raised heart rate, shallow breathing, dry mouth, sheer panic. So much so that the claustrophobia started to ruin my life, and it got to such a level by 2007 that I daren't lock the door in a public loo, I couldn't go into my cellar or garage, I was unable to travel in the back of two-door saloon cars, unable to go into large department stores because of losing sight of the exit, and unable to use lifts or go on public transport.

It was my friends' wedding in February 2008, and they announced they were getting married in Mexico! I didn't want to let them down, but I knew I couldn't possibly go because of my claustrophobia on the aeroplane. I knew that as soon as the flight attendants closed the doors I would panic. It all seemed so ridiculous because I had flown many times before. I worried myself silly and decided I needed help.

After trying yoga breathing techniques, relaxation tapes and hypnosis, I was at my wit's end trying to cope with everyday life. Then I met Janet.

She listened to my problems and she asked me to imagine sitting on the aeroplane and seeing the doors shutting. On a scale of 1 to 10 I was terrified; all the familiar fears started to creep in. Then she started tapping on various parts of my face and upper body, and as she continued to tap, the fright seemed to diminish.

Within 15–20 minutes both she and I were locked in a small understairs cupboard in my house and I was wondering what on earth I'd been so frightened of. I wasn't going to die!

When we came out of the cupboard (that sounds stupid now when I say it) she asked me if anything significant had happened in 2002. I said my mother had died. She then continued to tap in a slightly different way while I was thinking of things that made me sad about my mother. I cried, but afterwards it felt like a weight had been lifted off my shoulders, and since that day I have only had tears of joy thinking about my mother. I am also completely cured of my claustrophobia.

The day I met Janet was the day my life turned back around. I hate to think what sort of a state I'd be in if I hadn't taken the plunge and contacted her. I'm not a big believer in miracles, but that's the only word I can think of to describe what happened that day.

Janet, you have my everlasting gratitude for helping with the claustrophobia, but the biggest gift you have given me is teaching me techniques that can be used in other areas of my life too, and I even feel able to help others by showing them, too.

Eliminating Anxiety

Anxiety can be anything from an irritation to a debilitating fear. Many phobias are based on anxiety, and often a phobic has naturally anxious behaviour patterns. In the UK the National Phobic Society has now been renamed Anxiety UK.

Some of the physical symptoms of anxiety include:

- **tension in your muscles**
- **headache and unexplained aches and pains**
- **upset stomach – nausea**
- **diarrhoea**
- **erratic heart rate**
- **high blood pressure**
- **excessive sweating or flushing**
- **ongoing negative thoughts and feelings**
- **overreaction to minor unpleasant events.**

Some people know exactly what has made them anxious, others have no idea. As a therapist I have found that people who experience anxiety 24/7 generally either have a very full 'emotional barrel' or they have a high level of IETs (toxins).

In order to 'do' anxiety, you need to process information in a certain way – that is, in a different way to when you 'do' happy. Once you have eliminated your anxiety, then you can continue to use the tapping and other techniques described below to learn to create new ways of thinking and behaving every day.

Letting Go of Your Anxiety

Some people choose to keep their anxiety as they believe it keeps them safe, as is the case with many phobics: you must trust your natural instincts to keep you safe, these are in no way inhibited when you remove your anxiety. We are all born with a 'flight or fight' response: this is a series of metabolic and chemical changes that occur when we are in danger, such as dilated pupils, increased blood flow and heart rate, etc. When we were hunter-gatherers we needed this response to give us extra energy to run, either to catch our dinner or to run away to stop us from being some animal's dinner! When you have ongoing anxiety, then you are in a permanent state of fight or flight. This puts enormous strain on your endocrine (hormonal) system and can lead to reduced physical health and disease, which makes you feel more anxious and 'stressed'. Eliminating anxieties can be of *huge* benefit to your health. The TFT techniques I will show you can help you on a daily basis so that, even after you have eliminated your anxiety, you will have the tools necessary to use if or when you are in potentially 'anxious' situations in the future.

Keep in mind that some anxiety is not just normal, it is helpful: you ask any athlete if they would give up their anxiety when they are at the starting blocks and they will say no, they use it to their best advantage. I have worked with many actors, and all of them say that the day they stop feeling a bit anxious is the day they stop caring about their performance. They don't want to completely stop feeling anxious, they just want to get rid of the excess anxiety which, rather than helping them raise their game and deliver a great performance, actually holds them back in fear. This is the anxiety you can eliminate.

The treatment for eliminating anxiety is similar to the treatment for phobias. Often there is an underlying event or series of events that has led to the anxiety. Follow the procedure carefully, referring back to earlier chapters if you need to. Make sure you are somewhere quiet where you can concentrate and focus totally on what you are doing. Think of this as a proper treatment or therapy session. I would not treat you in a snatched 5 minutes between tasks, so allow yourself time so you can do this properly for yourself. It may take anything from 20 minutes to an hour, depending on your level of anxiety or how many things make you anxious; and you may wish to repeat the procedure another time to reinforce all you have changed. Take as much time as you need, as often as you need.

It is important that you are in a space where you feel safe and secure.

Now go to that place deep inside yourself and give yourself a message of appreciation. Maybe now you can give yourself permission to let go of all those things you have carried around that are no longer of use. Bid them a fond farewell. Let them go, and be in touch with things you have that fit you well right now. Give yourself permission to add that which you need.

'With your message of appreciation to yourself, you can now be ready for whatever you are going to learn today.'
Virginia Satir

Steps 1–4

Ask yourself these questions, take an SUD reading and write your answers down.

Step 1

What is the thing you are most anxious of?

Step 2a

When was the first time you had this anxiety?

Step 2b

What were the emotions you experienced at this time?

The Treatment

Now you have taken an accurate history, the treatment can begin.

Look at Steps 2a and 2b. Think about the first time you felt this anxiety and get 'in the thought field' of the memory. This is a traumatic memory and, in TFT terms, is treated as such in order to be eliminated.

Choose the sequence from those shown below that best fits your emotions. If you do not see one that describes your emotions here, go back to the table on page 107 and choose the most appropriate algorithm.

Basic trauma with anxiety

eb   e   a   c   9g   sq

Trauma with rage

eb   e   a   c   oe   c   9g   sq

_or_

eb oe e   a   c   9g sq

Trauma with anger

eb e   a   c   tf   c   9g sq

_or_

eb tf   e   a   c   9g sq

Trauma with embarrassment or shame

eb e   a   c   un   ul   c   9g sq

Trauma with sadness

eb e   a   c   g50 c   9g sq

_or_

eb g50 e   a   c   9g sq

Having chosen the right sequence for you, tune in to the exact thought field, think about the first anxious or stressful event that was the cause or the beginning of your anxiety. For this example I will use the basic trauma algorithm, but if you want to select a different one, simply use that sequence instead.

The Rules

1. **Tune in to the thought field and check the SUD. If it's different from before, write it down.**
2. **Treat as if there were a reversal and tap the side of your hand (sh) and under your nose (un) 20 times; then tap the sequence eb e a c**
3. **Take an SUD. If it is going down, then continue to Step 4; if not, complete the corrective treatment (see page 60) and then repeat Step 2.**

4. Do the 9 gamut sequence:

- Tap the gamut spot continually; at the same time:
- Close your eyes/open your eyes (long blink)
- Keep your head still and, moving your eyes only, look down to one side (R) and back to centre.
- Look down to the other side (L) and back to centre.
- Look down as if you were looking at number 6 on a clock dial, then move your eyes round to 9 o'clock, then 12 o'clock, 3 o'clock, and all the way round in a circle as if you were looking at every number on the dial, finishing back at number 6.
- Now repeat the full circle but in the other direction.
- Hum a few notes (e.g. the musical scales or 'happy birthday') out loud.
- Count out loud 1-2-3-4-5.
- Hum out loud again.

5. Repeat the sequence eb e a c
6. Take an SUD. If it is going down, then repeat Steps 1–5 until the SUD is 2 or less. If it is not going down, then complete the corrective treatment on page 60, and then repeat Step 5.
7. When the SUD is a 2 or less, do the eye roll:

- Tap the gamut spot continually for at least 30 taps and, keeping your head still, look as far down as you can. Keep tapping and gradually move your eyes forwards and upwards until you are looking right up into your eyebrows.

Corrective Treatment

If there is no reduction in SUD, then one of four things is happening:

1. **You are not in the thought field.**
2. **You are using the wrong sequence.**
3. **You are in psychological reversal (PR).**
4. **You have toxins (IETs) present.**

Check the first two, then correct for PR:

Try the first part of the corrective treatment first; you will only need to use the others if this first part (tapping **sh**) does not work. For more detailed information on corrective treatments, refer back to page 60.

- **Tap the side of your hand 20+ times (karate spot). This is known as PR1.**
- **Run your fingers along the underside of your LEFT collarbone from the shoulder to the centre of your chest. If you find a spot that is sore, then gently but firmly rub this spot using circular motions towards the centre of your chest, until the soreness subsides.**
- **Tap under your nose 20+ times. This is known as PR2.**
- **Do collarbone breathing (*see* page 62).**

When you can think about the time you first experienced the anxiety and the SUD is a 2 or less, move on to Step 3.

Step 3

Having cleared past memories of the specific anxiety, think about how you feel about the anxiety *now*. Put yourself in the situation now in the present time, either practically or by using props and memory access. Take an SUD.

Choose the most appropriate sequence either from those shown below or from the table on page 107 and repeat the tapping protocol:

<u>Basic anxiety/fear</u>

e   a   c   9g   sq

<u>Basic anxiety/fear with anger</u>

e   a   c   tf   9g   sq

<u>Basic anxiety/fear with embarrassment or shame</u>

e   a   c   un   ul   c   9g   sq

<u>Basic anxiety/fear with embarrassment, anger and frustration</u>

e   a   c   tf   mf   c   9g   sq

When you can put yourself in the previously anxious situation and the SUD is a two or less, go to the next stage.

<u>Step 4: Future Pacing</u>

Once you have reduced the anxiety to an SUD of 2 or less, then imagine yourself being unexpectedly in the previously anxious situation at some time in the future. Take an SUD and, if it is a 2 or more, treat it using the above sequences until it is a 2 or less.

Step 5

Now think of other things you are anxious about, and list them. Give each one an SUD; list them in terms of the level of anxiety, putting the worst first. Chronological order is not important at this stage.

Starting with the anxiety with the highest SUD, repeat Steps 2a, 2b, 3 and 4 for each one. If there are multiple anxieties you may prefer to do this in stages rather than all in one sitting. If there are just one or two anxieties, then you can comfortably do them in one session.

With anxiety, more than with most other psychological problems, Psychological Reversal (PR) is very common. In order to eliminate the anxious state it's particularly important to use the PR corrections every day, including collarbone breathing and tapping the side of your hand (sh) and under your nose (un) regularly throughout the day.

If you still do not experience a significant reduction in anxiety levels you will need to find a diagnostic practitioner or TFT VT practitioner (see Further Resources chapter) and eliminate your energy toxins.

Step 6: Swish

As explained earlier, the Swish can be used for a variety of situations where you want to stop a particular behaviour or response and change it for a new one. The techniques remain the same, but the content or the context of the images will, of course, change.

The Swish must be rapid and strong and you have to *mean* it. Use your imagination so that you can create really vivid pictures.

There are two ways of creating pictures in your mind's eye; for this technique you will need to use both:

1. **You can be *associated*, which means seeing things through your eyes as if you are *in* the situation; literally imagining what you would be seeing. It's your internal representation of what you see.**
2. **You can be *disassociated*, which means creating an image of yourself that you can look at from an observer's perspective, just like looking at a picture or a movie.**

You will need to make two pictures: one of how you see things the moment *before* you become anxious, in an associated way, and the second an image of you in the same situation but without the anxiety and in a disassociated way – in other words, how you would look without the anxiety. It is important that this is an image that you *desire* and want to achieve. Read through the process from start to finish before you begin, then do the exercise.

1. **Create the first picture, which is your 'cue' picture. That means what you see through your eyes, just before you start to feel anxious. Be *associated* – see it through your eyes. Then remove the image for a moment, but remember how to re-create or re-access it.**
2. **Now create an image of how you look and feel *without* any anxiety, perhaps feeling confident and safe, in control or**

maybe just relaxed with the absence of any stress. With this image, be *disassociated*: see you how you would like to be. Make sure the image is so powerful that it creates within you a real desire to experience this for yourself. Make sure you can really see it so clearly that you want to have it. Remove the image for a moment, but remember how to re-create or re-access it.

3. This time you are going to look at image 1 – that is, you with the anxiety, but in the bottom left-hand corner of the image place a small box which is the collapsed view of the second, desired picture, much as you would see if you had minimized a file on your PC.

4. Now *Swish* really fast – in less than a second, literally see the desired picture exploding onto the screen, completely annihilating the first, negative picture. Make the swishing sound in your mind as you do this, and imagine feeling the different feelings you will have as you see yourself free of the problem. Let these good feelings sweep through your body in an instant. Imagine feeling so good as you see this image of you as you want to be. Make it very powerful and strong.

Blank the screen, break your thought by thinking about baby green elephants, and then repeat stages 1 to 4 at least 5–10 times or until the first picture becomes so weak that, when you try and see it, it automatically disappears to be replaced by the positive image – or perhaps you can no longer see the first image and have already replaced it with the new image. Once you have done this successfully, hold that new image and anchor that feeling to that new image.

If you visit www.powertochange.me.uk you can access a free audio download that will talk you through this technique.

Step 7: Anchoring a Safe Feeling

Anchors can be used to support almost any TFT work, because you can anchor any positive emotional state you want to, and 'fire' that anchor whenever you need it. When I am working with a phobic, an anxiety sufferer or someone with depression, I like to help them establish a good anchor.

If you have got used to feeling anxious, when you take the anxiety away there can be a void and it's important to not fill this with new anxieties, but instead learn to remember that you can feel good for no reason whatsoever!

1. Sit back and close your eyes, and remember a time when you felt totally calm, safe and in control. It doesn't matter how long ago, whom you were with, where you were or what has happened since, just isolate the feeling that you had. If you cannot remember a time, then simply imagine how it will feel to be totally calm and in control. If you are a visual thinker, make a picture and then make it bigger, brighter, bolder and more colourful. If you are an audio thinker, think about all you heard, qualify the sound and imagine it in the best-quality Dolby surround sound now. Think about where in your body you feel safe, perhaps your chest, your tummy, just notice how you are 'doing' feeling calm.

2. Now take that calm feeling and imagine what it would be like if you doubled it. That's right, imagine you can

feel twice as calm. The feelings become even better, the pictures, the sounds and the emotions all work together to enhance your feelings and take you to another level of peace and calm and complete control.

3. Keep on doubling those good feelings until you are completely consumed by an overwhelming sense of feeling calm, and when you feel so good and calm that you are physically beaming, squeeze the finger and thumb of your right hand together. Think of this as a 'save' button.

4. Clear your mind for a moment and think of blue bananas, then switch back very quickly to the really good calm feeling and simultaneously squeeze the finger and thumb of your right hand together. Keep on doubling the good feelings until you are once again overwhelmed with feeling good (even if it's pretend, go with it.

5. Keep repeating Steps 3 and 4, generating the overwhelming feelings of calm, safety and complete control and happiness and then switching to another thought and then back to the good feeling, each time squeezing that finger and thumb when you achieve the 'peak' of good feeling. Do this at least five or six times.

The finger-and-thumb squeeze becomes your 'anchor', working as a switch, so that every time you squeeze them together your brain associates this with feeling happy and safe.

What Happens Now?

Learning to stop 'doing' anxiety is an ongoing process. You will need to tap daily to correct for PR, and use cb2 and the Swish and anchoring any time, any place you need to.

These techniques are free of drugs or chemicals, and can literally change your life. Allow yourself time to learn to stop 'doing' anxiety and start doing something else instead.

>>>Testimonial: Helen

I attended a session with Janet in a desperate bid to relieve myself and my family from the results of my nervousness and fears; I came away like a new person. Better still, I got an armoury of techniques to prevent a recurrence of those negative feelings. This success then led me to try one of Janet's training sessions to learn how to solve an old problem that I'd got so used to it had never even occurred to me I could get rid of it. I'd been suffering from a hair-pulling disorder (officially known as trichotillomania) for 45 years. The skills Janet provided me with enabled me to overcome it. I didn't even need to reveal to her (or anyone else) what the problem was; she simply taught me how to overcome it. It's been two years now and not only has the hair-pulling stopped, so has the compulsion. The freedom is exhilarating.

Overcoming Past Trauma

Traumatic stress is not technically a medical term, but refers to the ongoing negative physiological and emotional effects of a significant traumatic past event.

The vast majority of people with whom I work who are suffering emotional distress of one kind or another have experienced a past traumatic event. What is traumatic for one person, someone else can just shrug off; the way in which you react to an event is determined by your belief system and your values, and your ability to reframe any given situation.

'Everything can be taken from a man but ... the last of the human freedoms – to choose one's attitude in any given set of circumstances, to choose one's own way.'
Viktor Frankl, Man's Search for Meaning

Viktor Frankl was an Austrian neurologist and psychiatrist, and Holocaust survivor. In 1943 he was taken with his family to a concentration camp. Within the camp he worked to help fellow prisoners and try to cure them of their despondency and prevent suicide amongst the many who faced unimaginable loss and terror. For his own sanity he would walk into the yard and deliver imaginary lectures to people who weren't actually there. His wife and parents were killed; he himself was liberated in 1945. Frankl not only survived the Holocaust physically, he survived these most hideous events emotionally. He went on to complete groundbreaking research into behaviour patterns, his seminal work being *Man's Search for Meaning*. You might really benefit from reading this inspiring book.

People often ask me how I can work with so many people and listen to their dreadful stories, as I am known to be a bit of a softie (I'm the one who still cries at a Lassie movie and when people get kicked off *X Factor*!); I tell them I actually look forward to someone walking through my door with a huge trauma, as I know that in almost all cases I can eliminate it and they will be leaving the session completely changed and with tools to keep them emotionally strong. The other important factor is that what I do is not counselling. Even though I need a brief history or outline of the problem, my clients do not need to spend hours talking in detail about their negative feelings in order to eliminate them. I guess it makes me feel a bit like Father Christmas being able to give someone exactly what he or she wants or needs. I love watching my clients' faces as they get their desired 'present'. Now with all you have learned, you can give yourself that same gift.

Often when people come to me for one thing, I end up treating them for a past trauma as well, something they think they have already dealt with.

One day a lovely woman came to see me for weight loss. I am very well known and respected in this field and have many years' experience. One thing I have learned is that, more important than any nutritional or dietary advice I can give, is the understanding that people overeat for a reason. For some it becomes so extreme it's like self-abuse, although they would never acknowledge it as such.

I chatted to this particular woman for a while and it was clear she had tried just about every diet on the market. She probably knew more than me about the calorific content of any food you could mention. When someone has this much awareness and still overeats, there has to be a reason. I asked her to put weight loss aside for a moment and tell me what was the worst thing that had ever happened to her, as I suspected there might be some past trauma still affecting her. She then told me that almost ten years previously, three members of her family had been killed in a car accident. I asked her if she would like me to treat her for the trauma of that; she said yes. As I finished tapping, you could almost see the trauma leave her body; she was very calm and quiet for a while as she began to get used to not carrying the effects of the trauma.

I saw her again a week later and she told me that the anniversary of the accident had passed and that, whereas in every previous year it had been a very traumatic time, this year she had been able to remember fondly the good times and the memory of her relatives in life rather than in death.

Many times with people who come to me for weight loss, we discover that the reason for their comfort-eating is some kind of trauma or abuse in the past. I could fill a book with testimonials from people for whom I have cleared traumas. I really do have the best job in the world, and I am happy to share these techniques with you.

Carrying past traumas can lead to anxiety, depression, low self-esteem, physical illness and pain, and under-achievement. If you have past traumas, now is a good time to eliminate the effects and set yourself free.

You cannot change what happened. You had the trauma, and whatever it was it happened. What you can change, however, is how you react to it *now*. Each time you allow it to affect you, you are bringing it out of the past and into now, but its place isn't now, it's in the past – so keep it there! Once you have neutralized its effects, you keep the memory as wisdom, but its power over you is gone.

Use the following steps and set yourself free from the trauma that has held you back.

Before you begin, go to that place deep inside yourself and give yourself a message of appreciation. Maybe now you can give yourself permission to let go of all those things you have carried around that are no longer of use. Bid them a fond farewell. Let them go, and be in touch with things you have that fit you well right now. Give yourself permission to add that which you need.

> 'With your message of appreciation to yourself, you can now be ready for whatever you are going to learn today.'
> **Virginia Satir**

Ask yourself these questions, take an SUD and write your answers down.

Step 1
What is the worst thing that has ever happened to you?

Step 2
What were the emotions you felt when it happened? List the strongest first.

When you treat trauma with tapping, remember what you have already learned about the peeling onion effect: it may be that a particular tapping sequence eliminates one part of the trauma, perhaps the anger, but then a new feeling may emerge – sadness, perhaps. This is a particularly common pattern when treating trauma: any emotion can pop up at any time as you eliminate each layer. Each time a new feeling pops up, finish the sequence you are doing and then make a note of the new emotion and choose a tapping sequence relevant to that new feeling – and hold the new thought. Always remember to hold the thought of any particular emotion while you tap, and continually check for reversals. It's quite common to have to clear a PR at every stage when eliminating a trauma.

It may take just one straightforward trauma sequence, or it may take a dozen other sequences; there's no right way or wrong way to do this, just find the way that works best for you. If you can't find a sequence here that best describes how you feel, go back to the table on page 107.

Remember, you can only clear the thought that you are in at the moment you are tapping. If your mind wanders to another 'layer' or aspect of the problem, go back to the original thought and finish clearing it, then move on to the new thought and choose the correct sequence to eliminate that.

Now get 'in the thought field' of the memory. Choose the sequence from those shown below that best fits your emotions. If you do not see one that describes your emotions here, go back to the table on page 107 and choose the most appropriate algorithm.

Basic trauma

eb   e   a   c   9g   sq

Trauma with rage

eb   e   a   c   oe   c   9g   sq

or

eb   oe   e   a   c   9g   sq

Trauma with anger

eb   e   a   c   tf   c   9g   sq

or

eb   tf   e   a   c   9g   sq

Trauma with embarrassment or shame

eb   e   a   c   un   ul   c   9g   sq

Trauma with sadness

eb   e   a   c   g50   c   9g   sq

Trauma with ongoing fear

eb   e   a   c   e   c   9g   sq

Having chosen the right sequence for you, tune in to the exact thought field, and think about the event. For this example I will use the basic trauma algorithm, but if you want to select a different one, please feel free to do so.

The Rules

1. **Tune in to the thought field and check the SUD. If it's different from before, write it down.**

2. Treat as if there were a reversal and tap the side of your hand (**sh**) and under your nose (**un**) 20 times; then tap the sequence eb e a c

3. Take an SUD. If it is going down, then continue to Step 4; if not, complete the corrective treatment (*see* page 60) and then repeat Step 2.

4. Do the 9 gamut sequence:

   - Tap the gamut spot continually; at the same time:
   - Close your eyes/open your eyes (long blink)
   - Keep your head still and, moving your eyes only, look down to one side (R) and back to centre.
   - Look down to the other side (L) and back to centre.
   - Look down as if you were looking at number 6 on a clock dial, then move your eyes round to 9 o'clock, then 12 o'clock, 3 o'clock, and all the way round in a circle as if you were looking at every number on the dial, finishing back at number 6.
   - Now repeat the full circle but in the other direction.
   - Hum a few notes (e.g. the musical scales or 'happy birthday') out loud.
   - Count out loud 1-2-3-4-5.
   - Hum out loud again.

5. Repeat the sequence eb e a c

6. Take an SUD. If it is going down, then repeat Steps 1–5 until the SUD is 2 or less. If it is not going down, then complete the corrective treatment on page 60, and then repeat Step 5.

7. When the SUD is a 2 or less, do the eye roll:

- Tap the gamut spot continually for at least 30 taps and, keeping your head still, look as far down as you can. Keep tapping and gradually move your eyes forwards and upwards until you are looking right up into your eyebrows.

Corrective Treatment

If there is no reduction in SUD, then one of four things is happening:

1. You are not in the thought field.
2. You are using the wrong sequence.
3. You are in psychological reversal (PR).
4. You have toxins (IETs) present.

Check the first two, then correct for PR:

Try the first part of the corrective treatment (tapping the side of your hand) first. You will only need to use the others if this does not work. For more detailed information on corrective treatments, refer back to page 60.

- Tap the side of your hand 20+ times (karate spot). This is known as PR1.
- Run your fingers along the underside of your LEFT collarbone from the shoulder to the centre of your chest. If you find a spot that is sore, then gently but firmly rub this spot using circular motions towards the centre of your chest, until the soreness subsides.
- Tap under your nose 20+ times. This is known as PR2.
- Do collarbone breathing (*see* page 62).

When you can think about the time you first experienced the anxiety and the SUD is a 2 or less, move on to the next step.

Step 3

Having cleared past memories of the event, think about how your life has been affected by the trauma. What has happened or not happened as a result of the trauma? Write down your emotions and take an SUD.

Choose the most appropriate sequence, either from those shown below or from the table on page 107, and repeat the tapping protocol:

Rage

| eb | oe | e | a | c | 9g | sq |

or

| eb | e | a | c | oe | c | 9g | sq |

Anger and/or frustration

| eb | e | c | tf | mf | 9g | sq |

or

| eb | t | mf | e | a | c | 9g | sq |

Trauma and guilt

| eb | e | a | c | if | c | 9g | sq |

or

| eb | if | e | a | c | 9g | sq |

Embarrassment and/or shame

| eb | e | a | c | un | ul | c | 9g | sq |

*With past trauma, Psychological Reversal (PR) is very common. After treatment it's important to use the PR corrections every day, including collarbone breathing and tapping the side of your hand (**sh**) and under your nose (**un**) regularly throughout the day.*

If you still do not experience a significant reduction in anxiety levels you will need to find a diagnostic practitioner or TFT VT practitioner (see Further Resources chapter) and eliminate your energy toxins.

Step 4

Put your past behind you.

Earlier in this book I taught you about how we store time in the space around us. This is important; if you did not try this exercise earlier, then it is repeated in brief here now for you to do.

As this exercise involves accessing lots of memories, establish that the only memories you are going to access for this are either happy, or benign. For example, remembering what your house looked like as a child, or even cleaning your teeth yesterday.

As I ask you to think about memories or events from your past, ask your unconscious mind to make you aware of where you 'feel' or 'see' them. Start by imagining you are standing on a dial, rather like a clock face but with no hands, so number 12 is directly ahead of you, number 3 to your right, 6 behind, 9 to your left and so on. Each time I ask you to access a memory, simply be aware of where it is placed. We are looking for a pattern or a line. Although they do vary, for most people their memories will form a line (straight or wiggly) towards a specific number on the dial;

some may move upwards or downwards slightly as well, so just be aware of where specifically they are in space.

Start with a recent memory of something that you did yesterday.

- **Now think of something that you did or that happened a few days or a week ago.**
- **Now think of something that you did or that happened a few weeks ago.**
- **Now think of something that you did or that happened a couple of months or so ago.**
- **Now think of something that you did or that happened about a year ago.**
- **Now think of something that you did or that happened about 2–3 years ago.**
- **Now think of something that you did or that happened about 7–8 years ago.**
- **Now think of something that you did or that happened about 10–15 years ago.**
- **Now think of something that you did or that happened about 20 or more years ago.**
- **Now think of something that you did or that happened when you were a young child, perhaps a school memory.**
- **Now think of your earliest happy memory.**

Using your dominant arm, point to where in space you see, feel or sense that these memories are. Remember that point, and lower your arm.

Now think about your future. You get to play a little here, as you can create an imaginary future based on what you would like to happen, and it will work, even though it is a 'created' memory.

- **Imagine something you know or would like to happen tomorrow.**
- **Imagine something you know or would like to happen next week.**
- **Imagine something you know or would like to happen in a month or so.**
- **Imagine something you know or would like to happen in 6 months or so.**
- **Imagine something you know or would like to happen in a year or so.**
- **Imagine something you know or would like to happen in 2–3 years.**
- **Imagine something you know or would like to happen in 5–7 years.**
- **Imagine something you know or would like to happen in 12–15 years.**
- **Imagine something you know or would like to happen in 20 years.**
- **Imagine something you know or would like to happen as far as you want to see right now into your future.**

Using your other arm, point to where in space you see, feel or sense that these memories are.

Using the figure below, draw a line outwards in the direction of your past, and a line in the direction of your future.

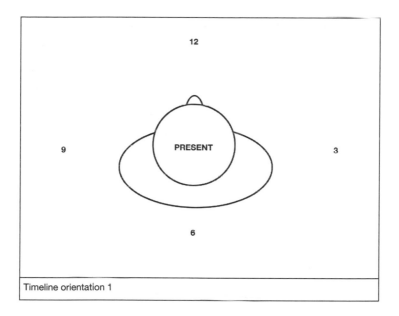

Timeline orientation 1

The best place for your past is *behind* you. And the best place for your future is *straight in front of* you. If you are not in this alignment, then do the following exercise:

Close your eyes and visualize your past timeline. See it as a rope, string, thread, pole, whatever works for you, but notice its place in space and its colour. Now imagine a safe pair of hands, or some invisible good energy, gently but firmly taking your past timeline and putting it *behind* you. Take all the time you need to do this properly. When you know your past has been placed behind you, is stretched out horizontally in chronological order as it happened, anchor it there and accept its new position. Say thank you. You may or may not notice a change in its colour. It doesn't matter, it's behind you now, for good.

Now visualize your future, and in exactly the same way move it and place it directly in front of you, and as you do so lengthen it and fire it out into the future so far that you cannot see the end of it. It's a beautiful, infinite horizontal line that you can see clearly. This line represents infinite possibilities.

Now complete the diagram as to where your new timeline is located:

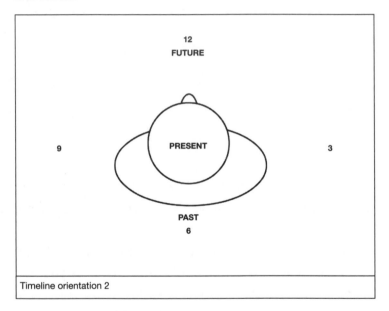

Timeline orientation 2

Now everything bad that has happened to you – is behind you.

Now you have put your past behind you, let's put in a safety gate. As with all NLP exercises, please do read this through carefully step by step before you then close your eyes and do the exercise.

Sense the space just behind your head, literally less than a hair's breadth from the back of your head. That is where your past begins, and it stretches out in a linear fashion right back to the day you were born, and even before you were born when you were just spirit. Become aware of this space and notice how easy it is to go back into the past, but know that it is not now. When you look at pictures or images from your past, put a box or frame around them to differentiate them from future images. That way your unconscious mind will know that these are images from the past.

Try it now, take a few images from your past – choose only happy ones for this – and put them in a nice frame so you know they are from your past.

Now move forward into your future and think about something you will be doing later today or tomorrow. Make sure there is no frame around this image, so you know it hasn't happened yet and is subject to change.

Now you know the difference between what is now and what hasn't happened yet, and what is past. No more confusion. Imagine you are floating up above yourself right now, looking down on yourself and seeing your timeline, with your past stretching out behind you and your future in front of you. Perhaps they are different colours? Perhaps not. If either one needs straightening out, then do that now. Notice your past goes all the way back to when you were spirit and doesn't actually have a clear starting point; it just begins to be there. And your future also has no end – it goes on and on. Even though you know that at some point it blends with spirit, it looks like a continuous line.

If you are a visual person, you might like to imagine, now, that all of your past memories are stored on slides, so that visualizing them is just like looking into a long box of photographic slides. Go back in time now and choose a slide that you would like to look at, lift it out of the box and see the image, notice how it makes you feel, remember in detail the event. What could you hear? Perhaps a smell or a taste? What is the feeling you get when you access this image from your past? Allow yourself to feel really good remembering this moment.

Now imagine that all the slides that contain traumas are empty – when you lift them out they just have a shadow of meaning and you can see only wisdom and learning on the slide. Perhaps there is just the word wisdom *on the slide, in place of any unpleasant image, or perhaps another word is there that shows you there is no representation of the actual event. What you have kept is what you* learned *from the event.*

In the form of a meditation, find yourself somewhere nice and comfortable, turn your phone off, perhaps put some nice relaxing music on, and sit or lie back and close your eyes. Spend a few minutes thinking about and noticing your breathing. See how many different things you can notice about your breathing: perhaps the difference in air temperature when you breathe in, compared to when you breathe out. Perhaps the rise and fall of your chest, or perhaps the sounds you make as you breathe. Spend a few minutes noticing as many things as possible and allow yourself to just 'be' your breath.

When you are nice and relaxed, float above yourself and look back at your timeline. Staying safely above your timeline, slowly float back over it and ask your unconscious mind to remove any images of trauma and replace them with wisdom. You do not need to remove the slides to do this, simply hold the thought of that time and think the word wisdom from the safety of your place above your timeline. As you are over happy slides, make these images bigger, brighter and bolder. Add a sound to the slide if you want to. Take a few images out as you go along, and enjoy them again. Know that you can look at these slides whenever you want to. Even though they are in the past, they are totally accessible to you any time.

Spend as long as it takes doing this; it may take a few minutes or much longer. Whatever speed you want to do this at, you can.

What Happens Now?

If you have been traumatized about this event for a long time and were aware of it on a daily basis, then you need to get used to *not* being traumatized. Make sure you correct for PR regularly throughout the day, and do cb2 morning and night. Also make sure you continue to put a frame around each moment as it passes. If it's an event you do not want to remember, simply remove the image and put the word *wisdom* in its place. If it's a happy time, then make the picture big and bold. Get used to processing information in this way and become first consciously competent at doing It, then unconsciously competent.

>>>Testimonial: Pamela – Parental Alienation and Child Abuse

I am a 45-year-old woman and after only two sessions with Janet, dealing with some very complex issues, some of which had been deep-rooted from the age of 12, I have been able to draw a line under many of the traumatic events that happened to me. These were things that occurred in my formative childhood years, which I feel had completely held me back from being able to feel true emotion. I now feel completely at ease with myself. These issues had been in the forefront of my mind for 33 years, and I had never been able to pass one single day without them surfacing.

Over two sessions we dealt with the child abuse first and foremost, followed by past and recent traumas to do with parental issues. I found the tapping technique initially slightly bizarre, but after following Janet's guidance I felt a distinct and immediate transformation of thoughts.

In the three months following my sessions, and also doing my own tapping, I can say with 100 per cent certainty that the techniques have been massively beneficial to my life. Mentally I have never felt happier and more centred in my entire life. Massive thanks to Janet for releasing me from those shackles … It works!

Boosting Self-esteem and Increasing Motivation

Many of my clients suffer from low self-esteem, and as a result they may underachieve in many areas of their lives. Self-esteem is, above all else, an attitude. It's how you feel and think about yourself and value your own worth.

Marilyn Sorensen, a leading expert in the field of low self-esteem and author of several great books on the subject, describes it as a 'thinking disorder' that has its basis in your responses to events in your childhood. Most parents are loving and giving and (speaking as a parent) do their very best and are very conscious of their children's needs. However, that is not always the case; I often come away after a day at my clinic thinking that some parents have a lot to answer for. If you think that your upbringing has affected you negatively, then another great read is *Toxic Parents: Overcoming Their Hurtful Legacy and Reclaiming Your Life* by Susan Forward and Craig Buck.

On the other hand, some children as they get older actually give their parents low self-esteem and blame them for their own failures, when in reality they are old enough to make their own choices. Children can be cruel to their parents, who have simply done the best they could. Whoever communicates negatively with you can give you low self-esteem, but only if you *let* them by validating what they say.

While TFT can eliminate many negative feelings and emotions, such as phobias, in minutes, eliminating low self-esteem is an ongoing process. Understanding how your brain works will allow you to make some of the changes you know you want to make.

We are all continually a work in progress, and the only thing that never changes is the fact that everything changes. You can choose to start to make those changes now, and every day when you wake up you can choose to make more and more changes using the techniques you have learned in this book.

Self-esteem is an attitude. What is your attitude today?

Validation

Self-esteem is either built or destroyed by your belief system and the amount of information you validate through your communications. For example, imagine I am with you right now and I am saying, 'You look absolutely ridiculous in that orange and green jumper with red hair and purple socks. You are stupid.' If I am there with you now, saying these words with total conviction, are you going to believe them? No, you are not, because you are (probably) *not* wearing an orange and green jumper with red hair and purple socks. Because the first sentence is based on a falsehood, you are unlikely to validate the second sentence.

Now imagine you are wearing blue jeans and a white T-shirt, and I say, 'You look ridiculous in those jeans and that T-shirt. You are stupid.' This time, the first sentence is true, so you are more likely to process the complete message in a totally different way: because you validate the first sentence, you might also validate the 'you are stupid' part.

Authority

Another key factor is the *authority* which you give the person delivering the negative remarks or behaviour. As children we have key authority figures, specifically our parents and, later on, our teachers. If these people, who have the privilege of having automated respect (without having to earn it), abuse their position and make negative comments and treat us in a negative way, then we validate this because of who they are. Perhaps surprisingly, some parents are genuinely unaware of the harm they are doing. They may have a misplaced belief that they are helping you 'become strong' by being hard on you; perhaps as a result of their own upbringing they genuinely don't know how to give you the love and support or encouragement you need or deserve, as they never experienced it themselves. Others are just outright cruel.

Of course, it's not just parents who create a sense of low self-esteem, it can be anyone to whom you give significance or authority – although, having said that, confident children brought up to believe in themselves and their abilities are far less likely to suffer low self-esteem later in life.

Patterns

The human brain likes to run on a system of patterns. We like what we know; even if it's not good we feel an element of safety in what we know. Because of this, children who are abused (verbally, physically or emotionally) often end up with partners who treat them the same way, as they gravitate to what they know.

In NLP there is a premise that the meaning of any communication is determined by the message received.

That means that when you say something that someone takes the wrong way, then the person receiving the message has changed the meaning of the communication based on their own processing systems. If I tell you that you look stupid because you are wearing an orange and green jumper, it has no meaning unless you are wearing that jumper. Then you may give it significance. This rule does not necessarily apply in early childhood, when the meaning is determined strictly by the person delivering the message. The child is an unwilling but passive recipient.

Think for a moment about something negative someone has said to you that you have validated. Now ask yourself this question: What if they were wrong? Write down your answer.

What does it mean now you know they were wrong?

Have a look carefully at your answer: What specifically does it mean? Perhaps it means you have wasted a lot of time and energy being anxious; perhaps it means you are much better than you thought you were? What does it really mean if you know for sure the other person was wrong? What opportunities might open up for you now?

How you communicate with yourself is the single most important factor in determining how you feel about yourself. Low self-esteem can be overcome, and often in less time than you might think, but it's not a quick fix as with the phobia cure. If I am working with someone with incredibly low self-esteem, it can take two or three sessions to eliminate the negativity completely and start to appreciate yourself and create a more compelling future.

Choice

The first thing is to acknowledge that you did not *choose* to have low self-esteem, but that you *can* choose to stop it *now*. You can reclaim your power. Whatever happened in your past is just that, in your past. Every time you think about it or allow it to affect you, you are moving it in time from the past into the now and giving it meaning and significance.

For an understanding of the importance of staying in the *now*, read Eckhart Tolle's books *The Power of Now* and *A New Earth*.

> *'When you are present in this moment, then you break the continuity of your story of past and future. Then true intelligence arises, and also love.'*
> **Eckhart Tolle**

When you bring past events into your present, you are likely to run the same negative patterns over and over again, get the same negative outcomes and then further validate the initial negative beliefs.

Working to eliminate low self-esteem is rather like transforming a rundown, overgrown garden into a beautiful work of art. First step – weeding!

Go to that place deep inside yourself and give yourself a message of appreciation. Maybe now you can give yourself permission to let go of all those things you have carried around that are no longer of use. Bid them a fond farewell. Let them go, and be in touch with things you have that fit you well right now. Give yourself permission to add that which you need.

'With your message of appreciation to yourself, you can now be ready for whatever you are going to learn today.'
Virginia Satir

Step 1

Write down the three most negative things anyone has ever said or done to you, it may be a specific event, a repeated behaviour or comments, note the feelings you experience when you think about it, give it an SUD.

There may or may not be many more than three events; if there are then when you have cleared the effects of these three go back and list the next three and clear those, and so on until the list is empty.

Using the most appropriate algorithm from those suggested below, follow the standard tapping procedure. If you do not see an algorithm here that describes your emotions then go back to the table on page 107 and select the one that best describes your emotions when you think about the event. Because they are past events they are all based on the trauma points.

N.B. When treating for abuse, then often the guilt and shame algorithms work well. Even though there is no guilt whatsoever involved in being the recipient of abuse of any kind, the unconscious mind somehow assumes responsibility for the behaviour even though it makes no logical sense whatsoever.

Simple Trauma

eb   e   a   c   9g   sq

Trauma with rage

eb   oe   e   a   c   9g   sq

or

eb   e   a   c   oe   9g   sq

Trauma with anger

eb   e   a   c   tf   9g   sq

or

eb   tf   e   a   c   9g   sq

Trauma with guilt and shame/embarrassment

eb   un   ul   c   e   a   c

or

eb   e   a   c   un   ul   9g   sq

Trauma with jealousy and/or frustration

eb   e   a   c   mf   tf   mf   9g   sq

Trauma with sadness

eb   e   a   c   g50   c   9g   sq

or

eb   g50   e   a   c

As you work through the treatment keep in mind the peeling onion effect: you may find that there are several layers to each event or emotion you work through and eliminate. Anger or rage, once cleared, often reveal a level of sadness, for example, so you may start off using the trauma with rage sequence and then, as the rage subsides, feel a wave of sadness. This is quite normal; just treat each emotion as it arises.

Having chosen the right sequence for you, tune in to the exact thought field, and think about the event. For this example I will use the basic trauma algorithm, but if you want to select a different one, please do.

The Rules

1. Tune in to the thought field and check the SUD. If it's different from before, write it down.
2. Treat as if there were a reversal and tap the side of your hand (**sh**) and under your nose (**un**) 20 times; then tap the sequence eb e a c
3. Take an SUD. If it is going down, then continue to Step 4; if not, complete the corrective treatment (*see* page 60) and then repeat Step 2.
4. Do the 9 gamut sequence:

   - Tap the gamut spot continually; at the same time:
   - Close your eyes/open your eyes (long blink)
   - Keep your head still and, moving your eyes only, look down to one side (R) and back to centre.
   - Look down to the other side (L) and back to centre.
   - Look down as if you were looking at number 6 on a clock dial, then move your eyes round to 9 o'clock, then 12 o'clock, 3 o'clock, and all the way round in a circle as if you were looking at every number on the dial, finishing back at number 6.
   - Now repeat the full circle but in the other direction.

- Hum a few notes (e.g. the musical scales or 'happy birthday') out loud.
- Count out loud 1-2-3-4-5.
- Hum out loud again.

5. Repeat the sequence eb e a c
6. Take an SUD. If it is going down, then repeat Steps 1–5 until the SUD is 2 or less. If it is not going down, then complete the corrective treatment on page 60, and then repeat Step 5.
7. When the SUD is a 2 or less, do the eye roll:

- Tap the gamut spot continually for at least 30 taps and, keeping your head still, look as far down as you can. Keep tapping and gradually move your eyes forwards and upwards until you are looking right up into your eyebrows.

Corrective Treatment

If there is no reduction in SUD, then one of four things is happening:

1. You are not in the thought field.
2. You are using the wrong sequence.
3. You are in psychological reversal (PR).
4. You have toxins (IETs) present.

Check the first two, then correct for PR:

Try the first part of the corrective treatment (tapping the side of your hand) first. You will only need to use the others if this does not work. In all cases, if you are using corrective treatment because TFT is not working, it is important to remain focused on the problem while using the treatment.

- **Tap the side of your hand 20+ times (karate spot). This is known as PR1.**
- **Run your fingers along the underside of your LEFT collarbone from the shoulder to the centre of your chest. If you find a spot that is sore, then gently but firmly rub this spot using circular motions towards the centre of your chest, until the soreness subsides.**
- **Tap under your nose 20+ times. This is known as PR2.**
- **Do collarbone breathing (*see* page 62).**

When you can think about the event and the SUD is a 2 or less, move on to the next until they are all cleared.

Depending on how many events or behaviours you are dealing with, do as many as you are comfortable doing in each session. If you want to stay with it and work through them all, you can, or maybe you prefer to eliminate one or two issues at a time. Whichever way works best for you, is the best way for you to proceed.

Step 2

Having cleared the actual events, just to be thorough, and to clear the effects of it through past, present and future, have a think about how each event/trauma or behaviour that you experienced has had an impact on your life since. Perhaps there are things it may have prevented you from doing or achieving? Think about the feelings and take an SUD.

Event/comment/behaviour

Feelings/emotions when I think about how it has held me back

SUD

If there are SUDs of 3 or above, then this time-phased aspect of the event needs to be eliminated. Using exactly the same selection of sequences and procedures shown above, repeat the tapping procedure but focus your thoughts on how the event has affected and is affecting you in the now.

Step 3

Once you have eliminated the negative past influences, then you can begin to work on increasing your self-esteem. The following tapping sequence is slightly different from the other sequences because, although we are eliminating a negative emotion, we are actually increasing self-esteem. For that reason the SUD scale of 1–10 is not always appropriate in its usual form (i.e. with 10 being the worst). In this case, write down the numbers as they are listed below, from left to right, and circle where you think your self-esteem is now with 10 being the highest.

1 2 3 4 5 6 7 8 9 10

For best effect, do this next sequence standing in front of a mirror: use the protocol as shown previously, including corrective treatments as and when necessary, and tap the side of your hand (**sh**) and under your nose (**un**) before you begin, to clear any potential reversal.

eb   e   a   c   un ul   c   mf tf c   9g sq

Keep repeating the sequence until you can experience a significant increase in your score.

As improving your self-esteem is an ongoing process, do collarbone breathing (cb2) every day and tap the side of your hand throughout the day. In addition, every morning before you start the day, look in the mirror and do the above sequence. This will greatly speed up the time it takes you to learn to feel better about yourself, and regain your self-respect and reclaim your power.

<u>Step 4</u>
Take control of your inner voice.

Be careful what you say – you might be listening!

We all have it, that internal voice that gives us a running commentary on our lives. You have probably never thought about how it sounds or tried to change it if it says something you don't like, but you can. You have complete control over your inner voice, in fact it is just a playback system that feeds back information to you which you have taken in and validated. Your inner voice determines to a very large extent how you feel and what you do. Your internal dialogue, your language and how you talk to yourself is part of your make-up, and if it is not serving you as it is, then you can delete that particular frequency and transmit on a much better one. It takes some practice, but it can be done. Try this exercise:

- **Go inside your head and count to 10.**
- **Go inside your head and count to 10 but miss out number 7**
- **Go inside your head and count to 10, miss out number 7 and do it in sexy foreign accent.**

If you can do this, then you have shown yourself beyond any doubt that you can control what goes on inside your head.

If you have low self-esteem then you probably have quite an influential negative voice. What does it sound like specifically? Allow yourself, just for a moment, to say something negative to yourself. Pick something that you say often and believe. Write the comment down and then listen to how you say it. As you do this, take an SUD on a scale of 1–10, with 10 being the worst. How does this make you feel?

Now think of a cartoon voice, again, as earlier, making it something really silly, perhaps Mickey Mouse or Scooby Doo. Look at the statement again, but this time imagine you are hearing it in your cartoon voice. Make it sound very silly. Stop reading and say it aloud, now.

Now take an SUD. If you have done this properly, then the SUD will have come down. If you use this new, silly voice every time you hear yourself saying something negative, it becomes less hurtful. As you get really good at this, with practice, it may even become quite funny and ridiculous.

Once you have perfected your cartoon voice, listen to it again and this time create an imaginary volume knob, and turn the sound down. If you are a visual thinker you may find that you can shrink the image of this character as you do this. Make it not only sound pathetic, make it *look* pathetic.

What happens is that your unconscious knows now that there is no meaning to this statement. It has simply stopped attaching any meaning to it; it becomes completely benign, just like the orange and green jumper comment mentioned earlier.

Now write down two more negative comments which you regularly use to insult yourself, and do exactly the same exercise. You can really get your comedy voice working here! Be creative! If you want you can add background noises, perhaps a crowd of other cartoon characters shouting your main character down, telling the character that he or she is talking nonsense. Or maybe you want to put images to it, making it very slapstick in true cartoon comedy style.

Now go back and read your original negative comment. Think about someone you love, a partner or a best friend, or perhaps a child. What would happen to your relationship with them if you spoke to them like that? Your relationship with *you* is the most important relationship you'll ever have. Perhaps it's time to start being your own best friend.

If you have ever trained a puppy then you know the best way to get it to do what you want is through praise and reward. It's the same with children: they thrive on encouragement and praise. In her 1992 Oscar acceptance speech, having been named best actress in a leading role, Jodie Foster thanked several people ' ... most importantly, my mother Brandy, who taught me that all my finger paintings were Picassos and that I didn't have to be afraid'. Just think how different her life might have been if her mother had said something like, 'Stop showing off, Jodie.'

I'd like to add a proviso here. This doesn't mean you will become arrogant and automatically dismiss anything and everything negative directed at you. It may be that some criticism is relevant, and although not put as elegantly as you would like, it may actually point up a behaviour that is no longer serving you, and that it would be good to change. The key is to process and differentiate between comments that *do* have validity and that contain information that may actually be used to help you, and other non-factual insults and accusations that are simply not true and not relevant, and are more a reflection of the person delivering them. In short, only validate comments that are relevant, and even then, make them constructive and use them to your benefit.

You can become your own mentor, the person who encourages you the most. In addition to that, surround yourself with people who believe in you, not people who criticize you or put you down. Unless you tell them it's not OK to do that, they will keep on doing it. More than that, if they hear you talk negatively about yourself, then you are telling them on an unconscious level that it is OK to speak to you like that, too.

Now you have learned a valuable skill, and as you practise it you will become better and better at it, and eventually this cartoon voice will become your 'default setting' any time you try and insult yourself.

Step 5
Put your past behind you.

Earlier in this book I taught you about how we store time. This is important; if you did not try this exercise earlier, then it is repeated in brief here for you now.

As this exercise involves accessing lots of memories, establish that the only memories you are going to access for this are either happy, or benign. For example, remembering what your house looked like as a child, or even cleaning your teeth yesterday.

As I ask you to think about memories or events from your past, ask your unconscious mind to make you aware of where you 'feel' or 'see' them. Start by imagining you are standing on a dial, rather like a clock face but with no hands, so number 12 is directly ahead of you, number 3 to your right, 6 behind, 9 to your left and so on. Each time I ask you to access a memory, simply be aware of where it is placed. We are looking for a pattern or a line. Although they do vary, for most people their memories will form a line (straight or wiggly) towards a specific number on the dial; some may move upwards or downwards slightly as well, so just be aware of where specifically they are in space.

Start with a recent memory of something that you did yesterday.

- **Now think of something that you did or that happened a few days or a week ago.**
- **Now think of something that you did or that happened a few weeks ago.**
- **Now think of something that you did or that happened a couple of months or so ago.**

- Now think of something that you did or that happened about a year ago.
- Now think of something that you did or that happened about 2–3 years ago.
- Now think of something that you did or that happened about 7–8 years ago.
- Now think of something that you did or that happened about 10–15 years ago.
- Now think of something that you did or that happened about 20 or more years ago.
- Now think of something that you did or that happened when you were a young child, perhaps a school memory.
- Now think of your earliest happy memory.

Using your dominant arm, point to where in space you see, feel or sense that these memories are. Remember that point, and lower your arm.

Now think about your future. You get to play a little here, as you can create an imaginary future based on what you would like to happen, and it will work, even though it is a 'created' memory.

- Imagine something you know or would like to happen tomorrow.
- Imagine something you know or would like to happen next week.
- Imagine something you know or would like to happen in a month or so.
- Imagine something you know or would like to happen in 6 months or so.

- Imagine something you know or would like to happen in a year or so.
- Imagine something you know or would like to happen in 2–3 years.
- Imagine something you know or would like to happen in 5–7 years.
- Imagine something you know or would like to happen in 12–15 years.
- Imagine something you know or would like to happen in 20 years.
- Imagine something you know or would like to happen as far as you want to see right now into your future.

Using your other arm, point to where in space you see, feel or sense that these memories are.

Using the figure below, draw a line outwards in the direction of your past, and a line in the direction of your future.

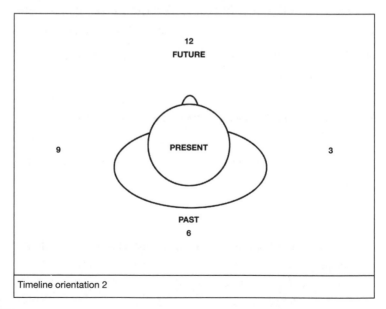

Timeline orientation 2

The best place for your past is *behind* you. And the best place for your future is *straight in front of* you. If you are not in this alignment, then do the following exercise:

Close your eyes and visualize your past timeline. See it as a rope, string, thread, pole, whatever works for you, but notice its place in space and its colour. Now imagine a safe pair of hands, or some invisible good energy, gently but firmly taking your past timeline and putting it *behind* you. Take all the time you need to do this properly. When you know your past has been placed behind you, is stretched out horizontally in chronological order as it happened, anchor it there and accept its new position. Say thank you. You may or may not notice a change in its colour. It doesn't matter, it's behind you now, for good.

Now visualize your future, and in exactly the same way move it and place it directly in front of you, and as you do so lengthen it and fire it out into the future so far that you cannot see the end of it. It's a beautiful, infinite horizontal line that you can see clearly. This line represents infinite possibilities.

Now complete the diagram as to where your new timeline is located:

Now everything bad that has happened to you – is behind you.

Now you have put your past behind you, let's put in a safety gate. As with all NLP exercises, please do read this through carefully step by step before you then close your eyes and do the exercise.

Sense the space just behind your head, literally less than a hair's breadth from the back of your head. That is where your past begins, and it stretches out in a linear fashion right back to the day you were born, and even before you were born when you were just spirit. Become aware of this space and notice how easy it is to go back into the past, but know that it is not now. When you look at pictures or images from your past, put a box or frame around them to differentiate them from future images. That way your unconscious mind will know that these are images from the past.

Try it now; take a few images from your past, choose only happy ones for this, and put them in a nice frame so you know they are from your past. Now move forward into your future and think about something you will be doing later today or tomorrow. Make sure there is NO frame around this image, so you know it hasn't happened yet and is subject to change.

Now you know the difference between what is now and what hasn't happened yet, and what is past. No more confusion. Imagine you are floating up above yourself right now, looking down on yourself and seeing your timeline, with your past stretching out behind you and your future in front of you. Perhaps they are different colours? Perhaps not. If either one needs straightening out, then do that now. Notice your past goes all the way back to before you had a physical form, to when you were spirit, and doesn't actually have a clear starting point, it just begins to be there. Your future also has no end – it goes on and on, even though you know at some point it blends with spirit, it looks like a continuous line.

If you are a visual person, you might like to imagine, now, that all of your past memories are stored on slides, so that visualizing them is just like looking into a long box of photographic slides. Slides can either represent a period of time, say an hour or a day or even longer, or just a short moment in time. Go back in time now and choose a happy slide that you would like to look at. Lift it out of the box and see the image. Notice how it makes you feel. Remember in detail the event: what could you hear? Perhaps a smell or a taste? What is the feeling you get when you access this image from your past? Allow yourself to feel really good remembering this moment.

In the form of a meditation, find yourself somewhere nice and comfortable, turn your phone off, perhaps put some nice relaxing music on, and sit or lie back and close your eyes. Spend a few minutes thinking about and noticing your breathing. See how many different things you can notice about your breathing: perhaps the difference in air temperature when you breathe in, compared to when you breathe out. Perhaps the rise and fall of your chest, or perhaps the sounds you make as you breathe. Spend a few minutes noticing as many things as possible and allow yourself to just 'be' your breath.

Start at the present moment looking down on yourself now. Then float steadily backwards along the entire length of your timeline, and as you do so, notice all the slides or times when you did not feel good enough. As you come across these slides, change them into black and white and make them very dim, so that when you pass over them or lift them out to look at them, they just have a shadow of meaning. Know that you can keep all the wisdom from the event; you have learned what you needed to learn and there's no need to revisit the pain, it can be deleted and removed now. Some things are good to remember to forget.

As you float over your happy slides, make these images bigger, brighter and bolder. Add a sound to the slide if you want to. Take a few images out as you go along, and enjoy them again. Know that you can look at these slides whenever you want to. Even though they are in the past, they are totally accessible to you any time. Spend as long as it takes doing this; it may take a few minutes or much longer. Whatever speed you want to do this at, you can.

There are many meditations that you can do, and the techniques you have already learned can be used to your best advantage so that you can rebuild your self-esteem and self-worth. Here are some examples of how you can adapt the exercises you have learned:

Anchoring

Find a time when you felt really good about yourself. It doesn't matter how far you have to go back in time, or even if you need to imagine how it would feel to feel good about yourself. Take this feeling, notice where it is in your body and make it bigger and bigger, and using the techniques described on page 136, anchor this feeling and 'fire' this anchor several times a day.

The Swish

Make your first cue picture an image of you when you had low self-esteem. How would you have reacted in a particular situation? Make your second picture a completely new vision of how you will look with a sense of pride and self-worth. Notice what is different about this picture and make it highly desirable. Using the techniques described on page 140,

Swish the pictures repeatedly until you cannot access that first, negative cue picture.

What Happens Now?

You are a work in progress, as we all are. Invest in and work on your relationship with yourself as you would your relationship with your child, your partner or your best friend. This requires effort every day. Stop being cruel to yourself, and introduce yourself to your new best friend – you. In this chapter you have learned some great techniques, and if you have already been using the TFT treatments you will have eliminated a lot of the causes of your low self-esteem. You will also have put all those negative events behind you, and you can know now that anyone who has ever told you that you were no good (including you telling this to yourself) was wrong. This opens up an infinite range of new possibilities.

Use these new tools and perhaps invest in some of the other books I have recommended, and enjoy the changes you want to make, today.

>>>Testimonial: Elaine

My childhood was my childhood. I knew no other.
I was one of seven children whose mother was tired,
ineffectual and had no understanding of children other
than giving birth. My father knew how to make children
but that was where he felt his responsibility ended.
He was in and out of work for most of my childhood,
but he was inclined to line the pockets of the local
landlords rather than clothe and feed his children.
I never knew that the scars of my childhood would
pervade my adult life.

Only as a mature adult could I recognize that the neglect suffered in childhood was the reason my head would hang in shame and I would feel a failure no matter what my achievements. I carried an aching sadness inside of me, and no amount of love from my husband or children was able to erase it.

I trained to be a nurse, learned all about psychology, read self-help books by the dozen, but nothing eased my pain. I was waiting to die and the sooner the better. This life with all its pain was not a place I wanted to be.

Then I met Janet and Sean, and my life changed. I learned about thought field therapy, this simple but amazing technique. I tapped away years of pain, neglect and rejection, and rescued the wounded child that lived inside of me. I was made whole. TFT and some other of the techniques I learned gave me the confidence and self-esteem I had never felt before.

I now have a fulfilled life, I understand myself and I know who I am.

I am eternally grateful.

Further Resources

TFT Courses and Workshops
www.powertochange.me
– For details of accredited TFT courses and other workshops using all the skills taught in this book, or to subscribe to the monthly newsletter

Personal Treatment
If you would like a personal treatment, email info@powertochange.me.uk

Voice Technology and Toxin Testing
If you would like more information about Voice Technology or Toxin Testing, visit www.tft-vt.com or email Sean Quigley: sean@tft-vt.com

ATFT Foundation
For details about the ATFT foundation, visit www.ATFTFoundation.org

Certified TFT Practitioners
To find a certified TFT practitioner in your area, visit www.atft.org

For More about Roger Callahan
www.rogercallahan.com

NOTES

NOTES

NOTES

Hay House Titles of Related Interest

Ask and It Is Given
by Esther and Jerry Hicks

Be Happy
by Robert Holden

Positive Shrinking
by Kevin Laye

Success Intelligence
by Robert Holden

Why Kindness Is Good for You
by David R. Hamilton PhD

You Can Have What You Want
by Michael Neill

You Can Heal Your Life
by Louise L. Hay

JOIN THE HAY HOUSE FAMILY

As the leading self-help, mind, body and spirit publisher in the UK, we'd like to welcome you to our family so that you can enjoy all the benefits our website has to offer.

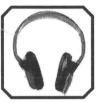 **EXTRACTS** from a selection of your favourite author titles

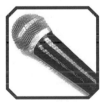 **COMPETITIONS, PRIZES & SPECIAL OFFERS** Win extracts, money off, downloads and so much more

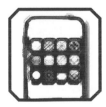 **LISTEN** to a range of radio interviews and our latest audio publications

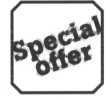 **CELEBRATE YOUR BIRTHDAY** An inspiring gift will be sent your way

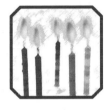 **LATEST NEWS** Keep up with the latest news from and about our authors

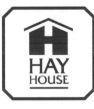 **ATTEND OUR AUTHOR EVENTS** Be the first to hear about our author events

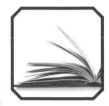 **iPHONE APPS** Download your favourite app for your iPhone

HAY HOUSE INFORMATION Ask us anything, all enquiries answered

join us online at **www.hayhouse.co.uk**

 292B Kensal Road, London W10 5BE
T: 020 8962 1230 E: info@hayhouse.co.uk